Democratic Dialogue
IN *Education*

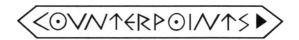

Studies in the
Postmodern Theory of Education

Joe L. Kincheloe and Shirley R. Steinberg
General Editors

Vol. 240

PETER LANG
New York • Washington, D.C./Baltimore • Bern
Frankfurt am Main • Berlin • Brussels • Vienna • Oxford

Democratic Dialogue IN Education

TROUBLING Speech, DISTURBING Silence

Edited by MEGAN BOLER

PETER LANG
New York • Washington, D.C./Baltimore • Bern
Frankfurt am Main • Berlin • Brussels • Vienna • Oxford

Library of Congress Cataloging-in-Publication Data

Democratic dialogue in education: troubling speech,
disturbing silence / edited by Megan Boler.
p. cm. — (Counterpoints; v. 240)
1. Critical pedagogy. 2. Postmodernism and education. I. Boler, Megan.
II. Series: Counterpoints (New York, N.Y.); v. 240.
LC196.D46   370.11'5—dc22   2003025195
ISBN 978-0-8204-6319-3
ISSN 1058-1634

Bibliographic information published by **Die Deutsche Bibliothek**.
Die Deutsche Bibliothek lists this publication in the "Deutsche
Nationalbibliografie"; detailed bibliographic data is available
on the Internet at http://dnb.ddb.de/.

Thank you to the Philosophy of Education Society who granted us
permission to reprint three of the essays contained in this volume:
"All Speech is Not Free: 'The Ethics of Affirmative Action Pedagogy'" by Megan Boler (2001);
"The Ethics of 'Affirmative Action Pedagogy'" by Suzanne deCastell (2001);
and "Silences and Silencing Silences," by Huey-Li Li (2002).

Cover design by Sophie Boorsch Appel
Cover image © 2004 www.clipart.com

© 2010, 2005, 2004 Peter Lang Publishing, Inc., New York
29 Broadway, 18th floor, New York, NY 10006
www.peterlang.com

Printed in the United States of America

Contents

PART III. MORAL AND PHILOSOPHICAL DIMENSIONS OF DIALOGUE

IV. DIALOGUE IN PRACTICE: RISKS AND BENEFITS

Editor's Introduction:
Troubling Speech, Disturbing Silence

In 1998 I was invited to be one of four speakers at Montclair State University on the topic of "Freedom of Speech vs. Freedom from Hostility." The public forum, scheduled to coincide with National Coming Out Day, spoke to a standing-room-only crowd about the tension between Supreme Court mandates for absolute freedom of expression in university environments, on the one hand, and the "Fighting Words doctrine," which expects universities to protect its members from racial, ethnic, and religious slurs on the other. I was struck at that time with a tension that remains unresolved in my mind to this day: how can freedom of speech be claimed as a functioning law of society when people are in fact individually and systematically silenced as a result of their identity and/or views? The lone educator on the panel that included representatives from the ACLU and NAACP, I conceptualized and argued for an "affirmative action pedagogy" to illustrate how social hierarchies confer unequal weight and legitimacy to different voices, making dialogue a difficult ideal to achieve in our classrooms. Just as affirmative action seeks to redress historically embedded inequities, so do I suggest that there are times when countering dominant cultural beliefs (especially within the abbreviated time space of a classroom) may require privileging traditionally silenced voices.

I presented a more fully developed version of my argument regarding affirmative action pedagogy at the Philosophy of Education Society (PES) Annual Meeting. Paper sessions at PES take the format of a primary paper and a response presented by a preselected respondent. In the response to my essay (reprinted as Chapter 4 in this collection), Suzanne deCastell contested numerous assumptions in my argument, including whether or not dialogue is an ideal to be pursued in classrooms and how voice is or is not tied to social identity. Over the next year, several colleagues took up the notion of affirmative action pedagogy in various written conference papers, and thus I saw the value of editing a collection on the tensions involved in fostering democratic dialogue in education.

The essays in this collection by no means share my idea that the price of freedom for all may, in some moments, require that dominant voices be strategically silenced. A number of the authors included here challenge this pedagogical approach. Nonetheless, each author in this collection is concerned with the profound ethical questions of how to create dialogue within classrooms that, like it or not, are microcosms that reflects the social hierarchies of race, class, gender, and homophobia that shape the larger world.

The subtitle, "Troubling Speech, Disturbing Silence" (thanks to Cris Mayo's brilliance), highlights the fact that what is said can be as troubling as what is not; and not only are both speech and silence potentially disturbing but easy assumptions about what counts as dialogue must be troubled and disturbed. The authors in this collection address such questions as: Should democratic dialogue be an ideal and aim in education? If so, how can it be achieved? How do we come to terms with the disparity between the ideals of participatory democracy and the realities of social inequality? When is dialogue a form of violence to the other? How do we recognize the complexity of silence as a dynamic element of dialogue, and how can silence be "heard"? If we abide by a commitment to freedom of speech, how do we facilitate the potential hurt and trauma caused by hostile words? Who decides which words count as hostile? What is the cost of policing words, even those that might at first glance seem to be words "everyone" would want to silence? Should rules be in place, for example, that correct for social imbalances by privileging some voices, or muting others?

While the authors in the essay do not share similar conceptions and solutions to these ethical dilemmas, each is acutely aware that voices carry differently recognized legitimacy. These authors are not interested in asserting political correctness as a solution to perceived social ills. Cris Mayo addresses the pitfalls of attempting to police civil discourse; Ingrid Erickson challenges Jane Elliott's model of teaching "blue eyes/brown eyes" and argues that reenacting racism as a way of experientially learning anti-racism causes undue trauma. DeCastell takes issue with how "affirmative-action pedagogy" as I define it might seem to reduce people's "voices" to an overly simplified "social identity," and argues that education cannot be obsessed with dialogue but must change its focus to how ignorance is produced. Resonant with deCastell's challenge to dialogue as a solution, Alison Jones questions the desire for dialogue and our faith in the "talking cure." Ann Berlak discusses a specific instance of her students' emotionally fraught reactions to antiracist views, and similarly Ron Glass addresses the inevitably risky work of getting one's hands "dirty" in engaging these volatile issues. Jim Garrison explores the philosophical dimensions of the dialogue as a form of violence, and Barbara Houston also engages a philosophical approach to conflicts of moral responsibility entailed in educational work. Huey Li Li addresses how silence has been oversimplified and must be understood as a complex and dynamic aspect of dialogue. Nicholas Burbules' Introduction summarizes each essay and poses provocative questions that should stimulate further opportunity for debate about education and dialogue in the contemporary social context. In sum, the authors in this volume represent divergent visions of what education can and should accomplish. While they share a commitment to education as critical inquiry and recognize education as an inherently political (rather than neutral) endeavor, the authors take radically different approaches to the thorny issue of how dialogue should be addressed.

The significant differences in these authors' political and pedagogical perspectives creates a text useful for sparking debate on the topic of democracy in education. Each chapter also reflects a unique disciplinary approach, drawing from fields ranging from philosophy, political theory, critical race theory, sociology, and feminist and post-structural studies. The diversity of themes that arise provides a variety of entries into the complex terrain of what constitutes democratic dialogue: hate speech, freedom of expression, speech codes, the meanings of silence, conceptions of voice and agency, "political correctness," appropriation of the other's voice, and "civility."

During the period in which this book has been produced and published, numerous political crises and legal landmarks put into even greater relief questions regarding inclusive and democratic representation in education. Most recently, the June 2003 Supreme Court ruling to uphold affirmative action in the University of Michigan admissions case underscores the ongoing social and political struggles for equality in U.S. civil society.

At the same time, the exacerbated expressions of nationalism, patriotism and fear cultivated in the aftermath of September 11 render the questions of freedom of speech and freedom from hostility more pressing than ever. The characterization of dissent as "unpatriotic" and virulent racism tied to discourses of national security radically impact the educational climate in the U.S. and in other nations as well:

- a backlash to academic freedom, manifest in the silencing of critical inquiry through such means as the website Campus Watch that profiles professors considered a "threat"
- community leaders and administrators directing students and teachers in K–12 schools not to discuss the U.S. invasion of Afghanistan or Iraq
- the SEVIS Act,[1] which requires universities to closely monitor and track the enrollment credits and visas of international students, making it nearly impossible for international students to return home to visit family, and also regulating when and if international students can participate in research projects[2]

The cumulative effects of the erosion of these civil liberties has been to silence critical inquiry and free speech within many schools and college campuses. The fear of penalization is not abstract, but quite real. My campus is but one example, and in the year following September 11 one of my students from the Middle East was told by an international student association not to research anything on the internet related to 9/11, for fear of being surveilled and deported.[3] A search on the Lexis Nexis database reveals dozens of news accounts of public school teachers and students and college professors directed not to discuss the U.S. invasion in Iraq. Not only do students face academic censorship/punishment but they also face physical violence. Two other international students on my campus were severely beaten while being called "Osama," and racially motivated attacks are frequent occurrences at other campuses. Universities have suspended and fired professors for publicly voicing unpopular views. In sum, freedom of speech can in no way be assumed as an assured right within a repressive climate.

Given that the climate of fear renders it increasingly difficult and risky to engage dissident voices, it is my hope that this volume encourages debate about how educational spaces can critically engage views elsewhere silenced as unpopular. The devastating effects of silencing critical inquiry and eliminating the potential of participatory democracy are well-described in this passage from Milton Mayer's interviews with German citizens under the Nazis:

> What happened here was the gradual habituation of the people, little by little, to being governed by surprise; to receiving decisions deliberated in secret; to believing that the situation was so complicated that the government had to act on information which the people could not understand, or so dangerous that, even if the people could understand it, it could not be released because of national security. And their sense of identification with Hitler, their trust in him, made it easier to widen this gap and reassured those who would otherwise have worried about it.
>
> This separation of government from people, this widening of the gap, took place so gradually and so insensibly, each step disguised (perhaps not even intentionally) as a temporary emergency measure or associated with true patriotic allegiance or with real social purposes. And all the crises and reforms (real reforms, too) so occupied the people that they did not see the slow motion underneath, of the whole process of government growing remoter and remoter. (1955: 166–167)

Educators and scholars who wish to retain classrooms as public spaces of critical inquiry face a tall order. We need to continue to improve our skills in facilitating difficult and risky conversations; we must continue to theorize our ethics regarding how to engage voices so that differences are heard. And we are faced with doing this already difficult job in a political context increasingly chilly to voices of dissent. Those of us who have the privilege in academia of being more protected than others perhaps need to shoulder the burden of struggling to retain democracy as an ideal. I believe the essays collected here model some of the courage, self-reflection, and intellectual rigor we will need to face the challenges of troubling speech and disturbing silences.

Acknowledgments

I would like to thank Gregory Maughn who initially invited me to contribute to the Montclair State University Panel on "Freedom of Speech vs. Freedom from Hostility." Gracious thanks go to Katherine Allen for her sage advice on thorny editorial issues, to Cris Mayo for contributing the book's subtitle as well as editorial direction, and to Jennie McKnight for incisive and insightful assistance. I thank Trevor Norris for his scholarly and generous contribution of the index to this book, and Heidi Burns and Lisa Dillon at Peter Lang for their experienced editing and production. The authors deserve acknowledgment for the unusual demands of reading one another's essays in order to create a fruitful dialogue between ideas as they revised their contributions. Finally, I thank the many students who are my continual teachers about conversation.

Notes

1. SEVIS is the Student and Exchange Visitor Information System effective January 30, 2003 by the U.S. Immigration and Naturalization Service. For a good summary of its effects see the testimony of Dr. David Ward, President American Council On Education And Chancellor Emeritus University Of Wisconsin, Madison, presented to the U.S. Congress House Committee on Science, March 26, 2003.
2. The SEVIS Act is tied to the U.S. legislation of the PATRIOT Acts 1 and 2, legislation passed shortly after September 11, 2001 which erodes fundamental civil liberties of freedom of assembly, privacy of phone and communication, requirement of warrant prior to home search and seizure, and due process of public hearing and law. The PATRIOT Act allows U.S. citizens as well as legal immigrants to be deemed "domestic terrorists." See for example the archives of the American Civil Liberties Union http://www.aclu.org/SafeandFree/ (retrieved September 2003).
3. These events occurred while I lived in Blacksburg, Virginia.

References

Mayer, M. (1955). *They thought they were free*. Chicago: University of Chicago Press.

Nicholas C. Burbules

Introduction

This important and theoretically challenging collection of essays explores the difficulties and dilemmas of fostering classroom conversations about controversial issues, particularly those addressing questions of racism and homophobia. As any teacher who has broached such questions knows, these discussions can open up prejudices, bitter feelings, anger, resentment, and real pain, especially when some class members are of the groups most affected by such prejudices. Sometimes, indeed, it seems easiest to circumvent such topics entirely, or to address them in only the most anodyne terms, to which all class members can easily assent. Going beyond this, to explore the actual dynamics, motivations, and experiences that characterize these persistent inequities, almost certainly will make a classroom more uncomfortable and tense. Some students will not speak at all; those who do speak may not always express their views honestly; if arguments break out, the teacher may not know how, or even whether, to constrain them—perhaps a brutally frank (if contentious) clearing of the air is just what is called for. All of these possibilities present pedagogical challenges. As the essays in this book thoughtfully illuminate, it is often troubling when students speak, but disturbing when they do not.

At a deeper level, there are questions about the *relation* of speaking and silence: How does the speaking of some students have the effect of silencing others (through intimidation, for example)? As a corrective, should a teacher impose silence on those class members as a way of encouraging others to speak? What if the teacher wants to encourage them to speak, but they choose not to? Can the very silence of some class members be an articulate form of expression (a kind of protest, for example, or a strategy of self-protection)? The essays in this collection shed light on these sorts of questions, confronting the reader again and again with the tensions inherent in socially committed classrooms, and exploring with insight the dilemmas of "silencing" and "privileging" student voices—challenging even the conventional understandings of what terms like "silencing" and "privileging" mean.

These authors write as theoreticians and as philosophers, but they are positioned here first and foremost as *teachers:* It is clear that each of them has struggled with these dilemmas in her or his own teaching, and the most striking thing about this collection, in my view, is the spirit of honesty and self-criticism guiding their explorations. Their views are not of a single voice on these issues, and important contrasts can be seen between their different ways of dealing with controversial subject matters in the classroom. The sorts of problems depicted here are never "solved," and there can be no single correct way to cope with them; on the contrary, I read these essays with a growing sense that *no* approach to pedagogy can avoid erring in some direction, that no teacher can have entirely "clean hands," that a commitment to certain groups comes at a cost in being able to serve the interests of others at the same time, and that as a result a reflective and conscientious teacher must make considered choices about the social aims and benefits that *can* be achieved in specific circumstances, and at what cost.

I think that most teachers will recognize some of their own doubts and questions reflected in this collection: What responsibilities do we have to shape the tone of classroom discussion, its directions, and its patterns of participation? What are the limits of those responsibilities? What are the dangers of doing too much, or too little, to control who gets to speak, and who does not? Moreover, as is consciously represented in my own inquisitive rhetoric in this introduction, which of these questions needs to be kept perpetually open, perpetually contested?

Another quality in these essays that will strike the reader is that, unlike most edited collections, most of these authors have read and thought seriously about each other's chapters. As noted, they are by no means homogeneous in outlook; there are critical tensions here, and significant disagreements. Hence, the effect is of listening in on *their* conversation, one that in some cases clearly precedes this collection; but now we, too, are invited to participate. This mirroring of content and design invites further reflections; it is part of what gives this collection its quality of dynamism, its sense of coherence as a conversation without closing off its conclusions—indeed, the book has no conclusion, and appropriately so.

In the remainder of this introduction, I mean to do two things. First, I will offer an overview of the chapters and their main themes. Then I will present a few questions and puzzlements of my own about the issues raised here—questions and puzzlements only, because it is not my proper role to put forth an independent argument about these issues and because in most cases I do not pretend to have better answers to these questions than those presented here. By highlighting these questions and puzzlements, I will try to suggest a few provocative lines of inquiry that cut across these chapters, engaging their own self-critical questions and in some cases extending them further. In the spirit of conversation guiding this book, and because of my own respect and affection for the authors I know here, such a participatory approach—while unusual perhaps for a introduction—seems the most productive way to engage these honest, challenging, and socially committed investigations.

II

Megan Boler's essay stands as a kind of keynote for the collection, posing the central question, whether and how far a teacher should go in silencing certain students' expression for the sake of foregrounding or "privileging" the voices of others. She terms this an "affirmative action pedagogy":

> a pedagogy that ensures critical analysis . . . of any expression of racism, homophobia, anti-Semitism, or sexism, for example. An affirmative action pedagogy seeks to ensure that we bear witness to marginalized voices in our classrooms, even at the minor cost of limiting dominant voices.

Unlike generalized principles, such as "freedom of speech," Boler advocates a more "historicized ethics," which looks at the actual circumstances and effects of these principles in practice. In actual classrooms, for example, freedom of speech for some students comes at the expense of others. Generalized bans on "hate speech," to take another example, fail to protect and serve the interests of the students they ostensibly protect. Indeed, even the norms of a common classroom and shared responsibility for education may have to be compromised in favor of "separatist spaces" that provide particular groups with a time and place to speak amongst themselves in a way only they can share. (Each of these major concerns is taken up by other chapters in this collection.) As with affirmative action in employment or in university admissions, any disadvantages borne by dominant group members in these arrangements is regarded as a "minor cost," necessary as a corrective to past imbalances and as a stage toward (presumably) more egalitarian relations in the future.

Like several other authors in this collection, Boler wants to question the general educational value of "rational dialogue," in two senses: first, because a "rational," unemotional mode of engagement will fail to allow the expression of feelings and experiences by members of marginalized groups that may involve raw utterances, "speaking back," even statements that (under a restrictive definition) might qualify as "hate speech" themselves; and second, because dialogue in the sense of an egalitarian, reciprocal, respectful model of interchange may be unrealistic to expect in many situations in a society divided by prejudices and imbalances of power—and attempting to do so places certain vulnerable individuals and groups disproportionately at risk. Instead of an abstract commitment to dialogue, Boler argues, "educators must commit to being allies to marginalized voices within their classrooms."

Cris Mayo is suspicious of attempts to silence "politically incorrect" speech. She challenges the efficacy of speech codes designed to prevent "harassment" in schools, arguing that such policies "are more intent on regulating words than encouraging learning and community. . . ." The attempt to silence hurtful speech does nothing to address the underlying attitudes and practices of homophobia, which do deeper and more enduring harm to gay and lesbian students; indeed, such speech codes may have the ironic effect of enshrining such attitudes and practices by effectively removing them from serious discussion and debate. Mayo's analysis here is a caution about the possibly unintended consequences of silencing policies designed to "help" or "protect" certain groups.

Like Boler, Mayo has no confidence in general rules and policies that ostensibly apply to all students equally, for in an unequal and unjust society "equal treatment" can be yet another form of creating disadvantages. (Recall the old saying that the law is even-handed because it prevents both the rich man and the poor man from sleeping under bridges.) Because school codes do not, and cannot, change the wider climate of hostility to which certain classes of students are subject, the apparent virtues of "tolerance" and "civility," *in fact,* take on the force of yet another constraint that can silence the students it presumes to protect. The same rules that prevent hateful speech against them often prevent them from discussing and asserting their own concerns. In this double bind, such students need to find new ways to act within and against these policies, in order to assert their identities and interests. Mayo depicts one such example, the demonstration of "Days of Silence," in which groups of students voluntarily, and conspicuously, silence themselves as a form of protest. As will be seen in other chapters of this collection as well, "silence" can take on many meanings, some of them quite expressive and not necessarily always a matter of oppressed victimization.

Ronald Glass begins his essay with an explicit statement of his commitment to a liberatory pedagogy: "[E]ducation as a practice of freedom entails constant vigilance, questioning, and challenging in the effort to make schools and universities positive forces in the struggle for justice and democracy." Readers familiar with the work of Paulo Freire will recognize phrases such as "education as a practice of freedom" throughout Glass's essay, and this Freirean view of pedagogy has two important elements: first, that liberatory pedagogy can never be limited to ways of constructing dialogue in the classroom, but that it always also related to praxis that engages social and political struggle outside the classroom; and second, that a commitment to educate/liberate the "oppressed" always also entails a commitment to educating/liberating the "oppressor." As a result, Glass is more inclined to promote classroom discussions that are (to cite some of his key words) "unavoidably risky," "volatile," "explosive," and "divisive." Along with others in the Freirean tradition, Glass places a higher value on dialogue.

Selectively silencing some students (Glass prefers to call it "muting," to suggest its relation to opening a quiet space in which others can speak and be heard) is in his view a perfectly acceptable recourse for the socially committed teacher; indeed, silencing is omnipresent and inevitable in any classroom, whether the teacher is aware of it or intends it or not. "Silencing is not the problem, per se, but . . . why and how it is achieved." Yet Glass also recognizes a tension in this pedagogy, since "A liberatory educator . . . would want to insure that even the voice of the dominant has some place in the class if only to subject it to searching ideological critique."

Suzanne deCastell wants to question the boundaries of this entire discussion. Focusing on the issue of bigoted speech and how and whether it should be silenced in the classroom, she argues, focuses on the symptom rather than the cause (there are echoes of Mayo's concerns here); correspondingly, the challenge of "changing attitudes and actions" goes deeper than pedagogical solutions can manage. Moreover, the idea of helping marginalized voices gain discursive space by silencing others is well intended but misses the point, she believes. In deCastell's view "voice" cannot be granted to others, it must be taken up, it must be seized—an idea expressed in Michel de Certeau's phrase "the capture of speech." For these reasons, deCastell is not interested in the problematic of how to foster dialogue in the classroom: it "doesn't in fact have the effect it is presumed to have," she says. "Classrooms are not safe spaces for 'dialogue across differences.'" As a result, affirmative action pedagogy "only intensifies the pathologies it seeks to remedy." The task at hand, she suggests, is better understood as an assault on ignorance, the ignorance that underlies and perpetuates oppressive and defamatory speech. In that assault, she concludes, it is "far better . . . to place our bets on the epistemic rights and responsibilities we bear as educators to combat ignorance, and to accept the risks we must take in their judicious exercise."

Alison Jones approaches a similar position but by a different path: What makes us desire "dialogue across difference"? What makes us privilege "voice" over "silence," and whose voice, and for what purposes? Jones in particular wants to question the "talking cure," the idea that issues need to be talked through, that airing such issues is a healthy thing, and that the solution to the problem of distorted dialogue lies in more dialogue. In all of these assumptions we place marginalized students at greater risk: open dialogue of the sort favored by some authors in this collection requires additional effort by these students to articulate their concerns (in a way that can be heard), to translate their ideas and experiences into a common language (which is often not their own language), to expose themselves (in a manner that puts them at risk of judgment and rejection). This seems to place a special onus on them. As is frequently expressed by members of such groups, what business is it of theirs to take on the burdensome task of correcting the ignorance and prejudice of dominant groups? Whose interests are really being served by such dialogues, regardless of who is doing the bulk of the talking?

Even more seriously, Jones suggests, the desire for the voice of the other can actually manifest an almost parasitic appetite on the part of dominant groups: while appearing to be an expression of concern and interest, and perhaps accompanied by admirable motives, the effect of such asymmetrical dialogue can be almost voyeuristic, and their own dominant status may be (verbally) challenged, but not changed: "Dialogue is based, however cautiously it might be considered, in a dominant group fantasy or romance about access to and unity with the other. This is the fantasy of a democracy based in consensus reached from rational debates across different views and groups. It is a truly magnificent, if flawed, romantic ideal." Speaking cynically, understanding the subjugated better in this manner could actually provide even more resources for continuing their state of subjugation and deflecting their *substantive* challenges to dominant authority. In such circumstances, Jones says, desiring separate, homogenous spaces to speak, and remaining silent in mixed settings, may be in fact an act of resistance and refusal by such groups to be complicit in dialogues that might expiate liberal guilt but do nothing to advance their own needs and interests.

Huey Li Li argues for the expressive possibilities of silence. Silence is not the opposite of speech; rather, they form a "continuum." There are different kinds of silences, and those truly interested in cross-cultural understanding need to take on the burden themselves of hearing these different kinds of silences. Forcing others to speak, to articulate what they think and feel in explicit words, is in Li's phrase "silencing silence," and she means this as a rebuke to socially committed teachers who believe they are serving the interests of those groups by "privileging their voices." Li is proposing a broader understanding of expression, meaning, and communicative responsibility; she also, significantly, illuminates the interdependence of silence and listening.

For Li, the socially committed classroom is often too chatty, too preoccupied with verbal dialogue to listen to its silences. In the rush to fill empty discursive spaces with more talk, real if subtle connotations are missed, and cultures that privilege silence (she mentions Navaho, Zen, and Indian yoga as examples) are effectively silenced themselves by an ethos that says, in order for you to be heard, you must speak in our way. In the same manner as Jones, Li wants to highlight the fundamental cultural asymmetry and intolerance of such an ethos. Drawing instead from the work of Max van Manen, Li describes different kinds of silences, and places the responsibility squarely on dominant groups to spend more time cultivating in themselves the capacity for listening (including listening to silences), and less on trying to "give voice" to those who may not want it.

James Garrison postulates that "violence in all dialogues . . . is inevitable." Similarly, Glass, who believes that harm (to someone) is unavoidable in educational encounters, Garrison therefore situates the responsibility of the teacher, not in trying to maintain "clean hands," but in "ameliorating" this necessary violence:

> Those who assume they can create safe spaces to sustain dialogues across difference in technocratic institutions must ignore the terrible asymmetries and inequalities of power perpetuated by technocratic rationality and its technologies. . . . Often, instead of attempting to construct safe spaces in their classroom, it would be better if teachers sought to grow in relationship with their students by rendering themselves vulnerable and at risk without necessarily requiring their students to do the same.

Drawing on the work of Emmanuel Levinas and Jacques Derrida, Garrison emphasizes the ultimate unknowability of the Other, which dialogue can never entirely bridge. However, he also asserts that "[a]pproaching the Other as if dialogue can occur enhances the possibility it will." In this conflicted space, Garrison advocates a "passionate ambivalence that strives to compassionately ameliorate the . . . violence" implicit in dialogue. Part of the intrinsic difficulty of this posture, he notes, is in the inability to read what silences mean in an unambiguous way: sometimes "silence signals ignorance," sometimes it means "pausing to think before entering a dialogue," sometimes it is "forced upon students by a totalizing discourse." Sorting out these different kinds of silence, as Li points out, raises thorny issues.

Barbara Houston also addresses the issue of conflicted responsibility. In contrast with several other authors in this collection, Houston believes that "there remain good reasons for attempting democratic dialogue," even though it is "deeply ambiguous and morally suspect." She concludes that democratic dialogue "is a fundamental activity of democracy. . . . If we discourage dialogue about these matters in schools, education risks losing even the possibility of transformative value, for everyone. Thus, I support attempting democratic dialogue about matters of social injustice in education, making sure that the challenges of it and the obstacles to it become part of the discussion."

However, in a discussion that problematizes even the very terms of its own difficulty, Houston notes, a certain kind of self-undermining paralysis can result, because when we reflect on the conditions that make democratic dialogue difficult, we all have "dirty hands" (it is interesting how often this image recurs in these essays). This expanded sense of responsibility can generate feelings of guilt and impotence; if we are all always complicit, then what can we do? Through a careful review of the notion of "responsibility," Houston acknowledges the difficulty of drawing simple moral distinctions in a "social political arena which abounds with tenuous causal connections between individuals and social harm to groups." Addressing such notions as "guilt by privilege," Houston challenges those views of empathic dialogue which suggest

> we try to take responsibility for problems of racism, sexism, or poverty by sympathetically identifying with the "victims," believing that through sympathetic identification we can better appreciate their hardships, sufferings, and humiliations and so are more likely to feel outrage and indignation on their behalf.

Instead, she offers a different strategy:

> I propose we see taking responsibility with respect to these problems as a matter of taking responsibility for oneself, not necessarily as a matter of identifying with any particular group. . . . I want to find a way to focus on what it means to begin right here where we are, in the present, in the midst of all our current resistances, conflicts, confusions, and tensions.

This "forward-looking" perspective on responsibility does not forget the history of past wrongs and harms, but refuses to be paralyzed by them; the sort of dialogue it fosters is one that looks at its own shortcomings and difficulties and problematizes them as issues within the dialogue, not as reasons to withdraw from it.

Ingrid Erickson focuses on the famous example of Jane Elliott's blue eyes/brown eyes exercise, made famous through the documentary "The Eye of the Storm." This exercise, which Elliott first used in her own third-grade classroom, has now evolved into the core of a widely used training program for adults, harsher in tone but still based on the idea that making people experience what it feels like to be discriminated against is a key step in transforming their attitudes about racism: "Stifling all attempts to object or engage in discussion, she silences her participants as people in American culture are silenced because of their skin color." The experience is intended to be "traumatic" for those who undergo it because Elliott believes that this is a necessary part of what makes the lesson potentially "transformative," and Erickson agrees that her work "is in many ways highly effective in addressing skin color and prejudice." Erickson notes the parallel with other approaches to therapy and psychoanalysis, in which experiences "that will necessarily be painful but that will not inflict lasting harm on participants" provoke the unsettling shock that makes profound change possible.

Note here that Elliott's reasons for silencing are different from Boler's "compensatory" view: whereas for Boler (and others in this collection) silencing is meant to counterbalance previously dominating voices and open up a space for marginalized voices to be heard, for Elliott the reasons have more to do with the effects this silencing can have on those privileged individuals who will get a taste of what others have been suffering. However, as Erickson critically points out, in Elliott's approach

> Confrontation takes the place of dialogue. . . . Because there is no dialogue in Elliott's sessions, the possibility of moral agency on the part of her students is foreclosed. . . . Her exclusive focus on racial prejudice overlooks the complex issues and ambiguous responses provoked by multiple forms of oppression and discrimination. . . . Elliott seems to be working within an understanding of identity that is based on a simple binary logic of self and other. . . . There are no shades of gray in Elliott's classroom, no means to move beyond the simple binary logic of oppressor and victim other than this temporary, painful role reversal. . . . Elliott's educational space is more theater than classroom, and it is anything but democratic.

We see this question of the educational value of letting members of dominant groups get a "taste" of what it feels like to be intimidated and silenced also raised in Ann Berlak's essay, much of which is dedicated to an account of a confrontation that took place between an African American guest speaker and the "mostly white" pre- and inservice teachers in a class Berlak was teaching at San Francisco State University. The speaker, Sekani Moyenda, had been a student in a previous class by Berlak; through a combination of role-playing, personal testimony, and "loud intense exchanges," Moyenda "challenged the students to see themselves as people who had internalized racist messages, erased those messages and their significance from consciousness, and, usually without their awareness, acted upon them." The other students in the class, not surprisingly, reacted with a range of responses that included defensiveness, anger, anxiety, and shame.

Berlak characterizes this approach to teaching also with therapeutic language. Drawing parallels with the work of Shoshana Felman and Dori Laub, and of Roger Simon, Sharon Rosenberg, and Claudia Eppert, Berlak applies the categories of "denial," "trauma," "witnessing," "testimony," and "mourning" that these other authors have applied to recounting and discussing traumatic events in their classrooms, such as Holocaust memories, misogynistic mass murders, and similarly horrible experiences. Like Jane Elliott, Berlak is interested in dramatic, experiential learning that, through trauma, shocks people into awareness and reflection; by contrast, says Berlak, "Much of what is taken to be 'democratic dialogue' is a repetition that does not disrupt the common wisdom. . . . It permits students to remain comfortable by reading stories of oppression and injustice as exaggerations and exceptions, and narratives of justice as the rule."

There is much more richness, passion, and thoughtful insight in these essays than my brief summaries can do justice to. In what remains of this introduction, I want to present some of the buzzing questions and provocations this collection has left with me. In so doing, I hope to suggest a framework that relates these chapters to each other and to a larger set of issues they raise: (1) what might be some of the unintended implications of an "affirmative action pedagogy"; (2) how the aims of a socially committed classroom might relate to other educational goals; (3) the complex interrelations of speaking, listening, and silence; (4) what it means to balance activist, socially committed, and other ethical values as a teacher; (5) contrasting views about social and individual change and how they happen; (6) the nature and prospects of a dialogical classroom; and, somewhat tangentially (7) the impact of psychoanalysis on educational theorizing.

(1) The first set of questions concerns the "affirmative action" view of pedagogy. The parallels with current debates over affirmative action generally may be revealing; the predominant sense of such policies is that they are an unfortunate but necessary means of compensating for past inequities, for the sake of attaining a more equitable future. Is that the sense in which it is meant here? Boler considers it a "minor cost" to silence (or, for Glass, "mute") certain voices so that others can be heard. Is it a minor cost? What other educational values might be compromised for the sake of achieving specific, admirable, purposes? Might such policies in the classroom engender a backlash of resentment, as other affirmative action policies have, that might actually render relations between groups even more toxic?

Do these authors see such approaches as a necessary, but imperfect, preliminary, and temporary stage toward achieving more open and equitable classroom relations, or as a steady state that will need to be kept in place for a longer time? Alternatively, as in the case of Elliott and Berlak, is such silencing actually regarded as a desirable educational condition, since it allows dominant groups to experience the same sense of unfairness and frustration that other groups commonly feel in classrooms all the time?

Similarly, is the maintenance of separate spaces for like-minded groups to withdraw from larger class discussions in order to focus on their own shared experiences and concerns, as Jones calls for, to be regarded as a stage in a process, a way of preparing them for the more difficult and risky project of engaging others who do not appreciate their experiences and concerns? Could it be a concession to the belief that such conversations are not worth the effort, that they generally do more harm than good, that it is simply not the job of subjugated groups to try to educate or overcome the ignorance of dominant groups? While the idea of separate spaces for relatively homogenous groups to work out amongst themselves their ideas, values, and concerns makes sense in many educational circumstances, without a deeper analysis of the multidimensionality of difference it can lead to a paradox captured nicely by an old Jules Feiffer cartoon: an African American character going to a men's group wants to meet in a group separately from the white members; but then also wants to meet separately within the black group from the heterosexual members; and so on. Eventually he is sitting in a room alone and says, "Now I feel empowered."

There is also a question here of when (or whether) students *need* to be "protected" from the utterances of others, about which the authors here disagree significantly. Framed too simplistically, some tend to worry more about potential hurts or harms to already disadvantaged groups; others want to emphasize the capacities of groups to shrug off these often-heard comments, to fight back against them, or even in some cases to reappropriate them and turn them back for different purposes ("capturing speech," as deCastell calls it).

Finally, is the breakdown of reciprocity manifested in affirmative action pedagogy justified? It may seem like a minor cost to some that certain students are excluded from a classroom conversation; but it may not seem so minor to them. Berlak says she tells her students that "reverse racism" is a misnomer, that "racism" cannot apply to "the verbalization of anti-white attitudes and the exclusion of white people from social events by people of color." The way she recounts this makes clear that it is a frequent response by her white students; can their reaction be simply dismissed in this manner? When students of color express intolerant, stereotyping, and hateful attitudes toward whites as a group (or toward other groups) what should one call it?

(2) This discussion leads to broader questions about what the aims of a socially committed classroom should be: To create dialogue, wherever it might lead, or to foster dialogues oriented only to specific, desired ends? To challenge and change the views of dominant groups, or to strengthen solidarity and promote transformative action on behalf of the disempowered? To educate toward the status of greater knowledge and understanding (which includes understanding the good and the bad, the politically progressive and the retrograde), or to promulgate specific values and attitudes which the socially committed educator believes will make society a better and more just place? These are not all necessarily incompatible goals, but several essays here implicitly highlight some and denigrate others; on what grounds, and at what educational cost?

Is it in the power of classroom teaching to change the wider society? The authors in this collection focus primarily on classrooms containing future educators, people who will themselves be influencing thousands of students. For this reason it seems especially important to challenge their blind spots and prejudices—speaking negatively, to minimize the harm they may do to their students, but speaking positively, to develop in them a commitment to justice and equality that they might represent in their teaching, in turn. However, as several of the authors here note, the problems of racism, homophobia, sexism, and so on, do not have their genesis primarily in educational institutions, and there is a danger of mixing symptom and cause; is it a realistic goal, especially given schools as they exist today, to place upon teachers the responsibility of societal transformation or is it simply easier to work on these issues with an audience of teachers, well-intended and vaguely liberal as they usually are, rather than confronting the real captains of racism, homophobia, and sexism in society?

At another level, what exactly is to be accomplished in such classrooms? Should members of dominant groups learn to feel sympathy, guilt, or shame? Should they gain a better understanding of how nondominant groups live and experience the world, or is changing their understanding superfluous? When members of non-dominant groups "speak truth to power," is it to get a specific message across (is anyone listening?), or is it more because of the benefit to them in asserting their voices and interests? Most of the authors here want to get past a sense of victimization for nondominant groups and the "politics of resentment," but who, precisely, gets to point that out? Can members of these groups only do so among themselves? If such sympathetic criticism is to come from the outside (as only some kinds of insight can), from whom?

Moreover, if the goal is not only to try to excoriate racism, homophobia, and sexism, not only to eradicate their expression, but to understand them, where they come from, why they persist, and how they work, can this be done without hearing the perspectives of those very people "infected" with them, and hearing them with something more than a sense of condemnation?

(3) One of the significant contributions of this collection is its reflections on the varied meanings—and interdependencies—of speaking, listening, and silence. Silence can be of many sorts; and if one takes silence as an indication of a problem, something to be remedied or compensated for, this depends greatly on what type of silence one takes it to be. For example (this might be worked out into a large, branching typology), silence can be voluntary and self-imposed, or it can be the result of external pressures and constraints; silence can be expressive, or it can be empty, unreadable; silence can be temporary, situational, or it can represent a consistent, even pathological pattern; silence can signify withdrawal from a conversation, or it can be an indicator of attentive, thoughtful listening. As Li makes clear in her essay, assaying silence and deciding whether it is educationally pernicious or beneficial requires attention to cultural and situational specifics, and cannot be diagnosed with broad, dichotomistic categories (either one "has voice" or one "is silenced"). A significant question here, then, is how can a teacher know what kind of silence she or he is dealing with? Whose silence is a cause for concern, and why? When certain policies, such as speech codes, that "silence" for the sake of presumably progressive purposes, actually have effects that block important conversations and criticisms from being raised—that end up "silencing" the wrong people?

Similarly, we are invited to think about listening as well. Several points are salient here. First, and most important, silence can be a necessary (though not sufficient) condition for listening. Of the many reasons discussed in this book for silencing "dominant voices" (to open a space for others to speak, to compensate for past monopolies on conversation, to let the advantaged feel what it is like to be disadvantaged, and so forth), this reason seems to be given short shrift: While people are busy talking in the classroom, or planning what they mean to say next, they are less likely to be attentively, thoughtfully listening to others. (Notice, however, that this is a justification for silencing based more on the merits of conversational interchange and how to promote it.)

Second, as with silence, there are many kinds of listening, and reasons to listen: listening to learn; listening as an expression of empathy or concern; listening as an act of obligation to others, growing out of respect; listening as an active process of perspective-taking; listening as a passive receipt of information; and so on. Here again, the educational benefits of listening, and of encouraging listening in the classroom, depends on what kind of listening is going on.

It is important to recognize that creating a discursive space in which some class members can speak does not automatically mean that others will listen to them; or if they do, whether it will be listening of the sort desired. So then there is another consideration: listening as a way of encouraging others to speak. How do we teach students to do this? This brief reflection suggests a complex interdependency among speaking, silence, and listening, multiplied further by the various forms these each may take.

What is key here is that the right to speak does not entail the right to be heard, and so from an educational standpoint, further questions need to be asked: How do people learn to listen, learn to *want* to listen, to what others have to say; might simply silencing (or muting) them actually make them more resentful and resistant to what others have to say? Peter Elbow (1986) describes two modes of listening, which he labels the doubting *game* and the believing game. Many academic contexts reward the first; but careful listening and perspective-taking require the latter. How do we encourage this? If changing the attitudes of members of dominant groups in the classroom is an important part of the purpose at hand (and for some of these authors it may not be), when can it be counterproductive to create a dynamic in which some students may blame others for the fact that the teacher seems to be favoring them—may become less willing or able to listen because they regard their being silenced as some kind of unfair punishment or (whether the teacher approves of this category or not) as a kind of "reverse discrimination"?

(4) All of these authors share an assumption that the purpose of the classroom is to confront injustice and to seek to transform society (although they mean different things by this). Boler says, in a passage quoted earlier, "educators must commit to being allies to marginalized voices within their classrooms," and it is not entirely

clear how this value fits within a teacher's broader responsibilities to educate all of her or his students as well as possible.

One way to frame this potential tension is the importance of teaching to change people and their political values and outlooks in a specific intended direction, balanced against the importance of teaching to communicate with a range of others and to explore certain facts about the world (an awareness that may or may not reinforce the political values and outlooks desired). What are the educational benefits of having a full and frank airing of views, even "politically incorrect" ones?

Several of these authors regard part of this socially committed approach to teaching as a matter of taking sides in their classrooms; treating certain issues of inequality and injustice as not up for debate, except in reference to how they can be overcome. As I read some of these chapters, I found myself wondering whether a teacher's role might need to be a bit more nonpartisan than this. In a situation where students (or their parents) are paying for the teacher to teach them, can any teacher make the choice that the education and advancement of some of those students is more important than that of the others? Does good teaching require a certain nonjudgmental stance toward student comments; not making them proof from questioning or criticism, but regarding every student's expression of ideas and values as a "teachable moment," and not simply as a target for the sake of making some larger point? Aside from particular interventions that are part of managing a class discussion (such as asking certain talkative students to hold back so that they do not dominate the discussion), can teachers set general, categorical rules about who can be in their class, who can speak, or who can speak on certain topics?

Of course, a strong response to this concern is that there is no "position from nowhere" in the classroom, and that teachers as committed individuals do not "put on" and "take off" their fundamental moral and political commitments when they walk into the classroom; that they should, and must, enact these in all that they do. However, this often seems to truncate what gets talked about, and which views are accorded a respectful hearing. The tensions here are real; I do not mean to oversimplify them.

A second set of questions raised by these essays concerns the somewhat paradoxical positioning of the socially committed teacher. Early work in "critical pedagogy" was very suspicious of teacher power and authority; the teacher's control over the classroom was seen as a reflection of the dominance of particular groups (especially when the teacher is a member of those groups), and so needed to be subject to critical challenge and "decentering" as the locus of knowledge; hence the emphasis in that literature on dialogical, co-constructed understandings in which teacher and student could shift roles and learn from each other. In these essays there seems to be a range of views on this score; for some authors, it seems that the unapologetic exercise of teacher authority is valid, even necessary, so long as you are on the "right side"; others recognize the problems, even the paradoxes, that seem to be inherent in doing this. Occasionally the argument seems to take the form that because teacher authority is necessary and unavoidable in the sorts of educational institutions we have anyway, and because the exercise of this authority always already does harm or violence to (some) students, all the committed teacher can do is try to redirect these powers to better as opposed to worse sociopolitical outcomes, and on behalf of those students who most need advocacy.

Perhaps this is so. But I wonder whether, turned slightly askew, this same rationale can yield a convenient rationalization for remaining comfortably within the conventions of teacher control over the classroom and the curriculum (even though the *content* of those choices may be more politically edgy and counterhegemonic). After all, the fear of "losing" control over one's classroom is something every teacher, at every level of education, experiences from time to time and—viewed from a distance—the various strategies for reasserting teacher authority under such circumstances can seem quite similar, even while their content and rationales may differ.

Finally, a related question is whether the teacher, with her or his particular identity, is a separate agent in the socially committed classroom—observer, facilitator, evaluator, instigator—or at risk herself or himself? If it is acceptable in one's classroom for one student to say to another, "Your ideas are racist (or sexist, and so on), and I don't want to hear anything more from your mouth," is it also acceptable for that student to say it to the teacher? What then? Does the teacher's sincere advocacy and commitment compensate for her or his own blind spots as a member of group X, Y, or Z? Conversely, are the teacher's intentions irrelevant once the discussion turns to positions and privilege? I know of one class where a group of students wanted to "withdraw" from the class and meet separately, not only from the other students, but from the teacher as well. What then? The teacher might want to Socratically turn such challenges back into grist for classroom discussion; but how can this be done without reasserting one's own privileged position?

(5) These essays also exhibit a range of views on the possibilities, and the mechanisms, of social and individual transformation. Several of the authors note that the actual origins of discrimination and hatred of some groups toward others are based in institutions and practices that are outside the control of schools; and that the manifestations of these in classrooms is more symptom than cause. Nevertheless, as educators we find it extremely difficult to give up the idealistic faith that social change can happen one person, one learner, at a time. Even when socially committed teachers talk about forming solidarity and engaging in "extracurricular" collective praxis as a part of the process of personal transformation, it is very difficult within the framework of our teaching customs and training to get past an emphasis on changing the individual.

Thus, in reading these essays we are brought back repeatedly to their (largely tacit) theoretical assumptions about how people change—and whose change is a focus of concern. Questions arise repeatedly about whether the reasons for critiquing the attitudes and privileges of members of "dominant" groups is primarily geared toward "empowering" and giving voice to groups who can gain in confidence and assertiveness by "speaking truth to power," or toward changing those members of dominant groups by challenging them through critique or by letting them experience what it feels like to be put upon. (Conversely, for the more intractable members of dominant groups, is the effect not transformation but simply getting them to keep their views to themselves, or to limit their overt statements merely to "saying the right things" in the eyes of the teacher?)

On the matter of confronting and changing retrogressive attitudes and beliefs, I think of the work of Gary Fenstermacher (1978), in another context, which suggests that it is not sufficient to change mistaken views (if one's goal is to try to change them), simply by criticizing them as wrong, or simply by giving counter-evidence to them. Rather, changing such attitudes and beliefs requires following the process and rationales by which they were formed in the first place, and that requires having some patience with hearing out views—up to a point, at least—that one might find deeply objectionable. Furthermore, it requires an act of imagination to ponder how it might be that people who are not fundamentally evil or hateful might come to hold such views. Certainly this kind of patience might be too much to expect from those who are the victims of such prejudices; but it may not be too much to expect from teachers. When these views are regarded as something solely to be silenced, or condemned, or held up as an object lesson for the sake of *others'* educational benefit, something of potential value, educationally, has been sacrificed.

(6) I have already broached the question of the kind of classroom one wants to create as a teacher, and the educational responsibility to maintain a certain spirit of shared inquiry within it. One important difference among these essays is between those concerned primarily with K–12 public schools, and those concerned more with universities. This difference raises key questions of age and developmental capacities, and about what can and cannot be expected of younger versus more mature learners; about what kinds of discomfort one can cause adult learners who are taking a class voluntarily (and who can usually walk out), versus younger students who are compelled to be in one's classroom; and about those who need to be protected because they cannot protect themselves, and those who do not.

The papers in this collection also illustrate another dimension of this question, which is how one views the population of students within the classroom. Nearly all the discussions here of classroom dynamics, of who needs to speak and who needs to listen, are based on a dyadic conception of part of the class as a "dominant" group, and the other as "other" or subjugated. The particular dimensions of this division (race, sexuality, western versus "Third World" students, and so on) might seem to be divided into sharp either/or categories, but on reflection these are not clear dyads. Moreover, any one of these bilateral divisions is not the only factor operating in any complex classroom, a point made by some of the authors here. So, when one is thinking about silencing a dominant group so they can hear the "other's" stories, which division is to be given priority? Is racial discrimination a more serious problem than anti-Semitism? Is there a problem with silencing a white, poor, working-class female student, for the sake of a racial debate, when the very same student might herself feel silenced or disadvantaged in the context of a discussion of gender or poverty? By what authority does a teacher prioritize specific issues as the ones that will govern student identities and positions in her or his class, relegating the others to invisibility or secondary status—are these necessarily the ones that are most salient for the students under these circumstances? A more multidimensional and relational view of difference, by contrast, would highlight the fact that dyadic dominant/marginalized, voiced/silenced, oppressor/oppressed relations are far too crude to capture the complex interdependencies of power operating in most classrooms, and would ask how all parties to an interaction of asymmetrical power contribute to that dynamic in various ways, and how they may all need to reflect and change themselves if they are to challenge it.

Finally, there is a wide range of views in these essays about whether fostering dialogue is a worthwhile or productive goal in mixed-group classrooms; whether it is part of the solution or part of the problem. Some reject dialogue explicitly. However, is the issue here with dialogue, or with particular kinds of dialogue; is the reason for critiquing, say, the model of "rational dialogue" in the classroom really just a basis for proposing an alternative conception of dialogue (of a different form, or involving some but not other sorts of people), or is it really intended to be a rejection of dialogue itself? Some of these authors seem to suggest that dialogue is simply not possible between people of asymmetrical power. This sort of self-fulfilling prediction flies in the face of the experience that people can surprise us with what they prove capable of doing, and that in some classrooms at least participants can rise to the occasion and produce honest, challenging, insightful, self-reflective, and self-critical conversations with each other, when they are given the chance. Might the skepticism that a teacher intentionally or inadvertently communicates about the nature and value of dialogue be a factor in discouraging students themselves from seeing it as desirable or worthwhile?

The authors of some of the essays here do not think that disadvantaged groups can benefit from dialogue with dominant ones. However, there is a different perspective on this problem, deriving from the anthropological distinction of *emic* and *etic* perspectives. On the one hand, there are certainly ways in which a culture or group understands itself (the *emic* view) that cannot be fully grasped or articulated by outsiders without a local explaining it to them—and even then they may never fully understand it because they are outsiders. At the same time there are advantages to an etic view because sometimes a stranger can see or recognize features of a culture or group that are so taken-for-granted by the "insiders" that they do not see it for what it is, or may not realize that there could be an alternative to it. While we live in an era that tends to privilege the *emic* view, almost to an extreme, it seems that the dynamic of *emic* and *etic* perspectives, within and across various lines of difference, may provide the richest range of opportunities for students of all sorts to confront surprising and perhaps uncomfortable things about themselves and the affinities they take for granted. The dyadic and asymmetrical model of classroom discourse presented in some of these essays seems to limit those possibilities.

In the context of these socially committed classrooms, who is dialogue for, and what is it supposed to be about: Is it a means of solidarity-building within homogeneous groups of the subjugated? Is it a way of sharing personal (or group) perspectives and experiences with others not like you—or does this promote a kind of voyeurism that abrogates personal responsibility? Is it a mechanism of persuasion, and can it do this without being "rational" (in some sense)? Is it an assertion (to the unconvinced) that racism, homophobia, and so on do exist—or is it intended to be an exploration of how and why they exist? Each of these views of dialogue drives crucial decisions about who gets to speak, who needs to listen, what can be talked about, and what cannot be.

(7) Finally, and briefly, I would like to note the theoretical impact of psychoanalytic perspectives, directly or indirectly, on much of this discussion, in three regards.

First, a substantial part of the mistrust people have in dialogue seems to be because they come from a perspective that doubts that what is being talked about (apparently) is what is really being talked about. Beneath the surface appearance of our statements is—on this view—a surging turmoil of unconscious motivations, emotions, and intentions that often belie our overt, polite expressions. Hence "rational dialogue," which comes in for some tough criticism here, is often not what it appears. Differences, resentments, fears, hostilities, power games, and so on, are always operating in the background. Several of the authors here want to highlight these other factors, to overtly disrupt the benign self-conception of "rational dialogue." However, it remains a possibility that a conception of dialogue in which these other factors are not ruled impolite or out of bounds could still be of value, precisely because it can be self-reflective about the conditions and constraints under which it is proceeding. Houston makes this point explicitly.

The problem, from a psychoanalytic view, is that because we might not be aware of, or be able to acknowledge and confront, such deeper motivations, it may not be possible to recognize and problematize them. Hence, the second point: that from the point of view of at least one of these papers (or from Elliott's point of view, which is critiqued in another of them), education is closely akin to therapy. Education, therefore, is regarded as a process of personal transformation (and not just learning or development), a process that depends in part on confronting suppressed feelings and beliefs that may be difficult for students to conjure up and admit to. Hence the strategies of teaching may need to include extreme interventions to "shake up" students and challenge them at a deeply emotional as well as cognitive level. For someone who regards as an aim of her or his own teaching to change the deeply engrained biases, fears, and prejudices of students, such extreme interventions are more than justified; for others, the broader goal of pursuing social justice just means that some students will be upset in the process—personal transformation is not the aim in such cases.

However, the analogy with therapy raises a few more questions. One is that therapy is normally either voluntarily chosen or mandated for severe medical (or criminal) reasons. Students enrolling in university classes, for example, may or may not be knowingly subjecting themselves to everything a teacher deems beneficial to them. Furthermore, a therapeutic relation is a long-term one, in which a therapist accepts the responsibility for follow-up and seeing a patient through the possibly arduous stages of coming to terms with her or his demons, and all that may entail (midnight phone calls, hysterical weeping, or whatever); a teacher who offers one class, in a series of classes the student is taking for other professional or academic reasons, does not have or claim to have this sort of long-term commitment and involvement. In some cases "therapy" assumes a model of what constitutes "healthy" personality and conduct; but the politically laden values of the socially committed classroom, whatever their merits, are not the same as this—it is not clear, for example, that a person who has racist or homophobic attitudes is necessarily a disturbed personality or "needs help." One's reasons for wanting to change them, or to help them change themselves, have to do with a different sort of value—and a value that the teacher prizes, not necessarily one that the student thinks is a problem.

Finally, to the extent that these therapeutic interventions require—in the language used in this book—"trauma," "pain," "harm," or "violence" for the student, further questions arise. Certainly experiencing these may be a necessary consequence, or even a condition, for certain kinds of profound self-discovery and transformation; and certainly teachers might inadvertently cause these kinds of sufferings to students even when they are teaching in more conventional modes. But to do so intentionally and systematically, with even the best of motives, undertakes a responsibility for which most teachers are neither trained nor licensed. At a simple commonsensical level, one might ask, "Who gave you the right to mess with my head?" Is it *ever* appropriate for a teacher to knowingly and intentionally cause "pain," "harm," "violence," and "trauma" to one's students, however valuable the educational lesson at stake? Do students need to be given the choice of whether they wish to be challenged and changed in these ways? In actual institutional settings, with grades, course requirements, graduation standards, and so on, is there a coercive effect in putting courses like this into the required sequence—in which failing to change in the appropriate way, or rejecting the teacher's agenda, or persisting unapologetically in incorrect views and opinions, could all have serious repercussions for students' future educational and professional possibilities?

Thus, in the critical and reflexive spirit of this collection, I add some more challenging questions to the mix. Some are echoes of questions explicitly raised by some of these essays already. As I said at the beginning, this is a brave and self-critical collection, taken as a whole, because tensions between the positions here are openly acknowledged and discussed. One could hardly imagine a set of papers so willing to pose tough questions to themselves and to each other. I do not pretend to have better answers for these questions myself (or if there are even "answers"); the book raises and honestly explores extremely difficult tensions between conflicting and equally important educational and moral values. The very title of this book, "Troubling Speech, Disturbing Silence," reflects the damned-if-you-do, damned-if-you-don't dilemmas that socially committed teachers have to grapple with. I share and support the commitments that drive these approaches to committed teaching, and hope to advance that project, and to enrich your reading and appreciation of this text, by complicating these matters even further.

Note

This essay has benefited greatly from comments and suggestions by Megan Boler, Natasha Levinson, Suzanne Rice, Fazal Rizvi, and Audrey Thompson. I do not mean to imply that they endorse any of the particular views expressed here.

References

Elbow, P. (1986). *Embracing contraries: Explorations in learning and teaching.* New York: Oxford University Press.

Fenstermacher, G. (1978). A philosophical consideration of recent research on teacher effectiveness. In L. Shulman (Ed.), *Review of research in education. Vol. 6* (pp. 157–185). Washington, DC: American Educational Research Association.

PART I

The Challenge of Creating Spaces for Social Justice Dialogue

Megan Boler

All Speech Is Not Free: The Ethics of "Affirmative Action Pedagogy"

All speech is not free. Power inequities institutionalized through economies, gender roles, social class, and corporate-owned media ensure that all voices do not carry the same weight. Within Western democracies, different voices pay different prices for the words they choose to utter. Some speech will result in the speaker being assaulted or even killed. Other speech is not free in the sense that it is foreclosed: Our social and political culture predetermines certain voices and articulations as unrecognizable, illegitimate, unspeakable (Butler, 1997).[1]

Similarly, not all expressions of hostility are equal. Some hostile voices are penalized while others are tolerated.[2] Hostility that targets marginalized people on the basis of their assumed inferiority carries more weight than hostility expressed by a marginalized person toward a member of the dominant class. Efforts to legislate against "hate speech" within public spaces cannot, in principle, recognize the differential weight and significance of hate speech directed at different individuals or groups.

If all speech is not free, then in what sense can one claim that freedom of speech is a working constitutional right? If free speech is not effective in practice, then an historicized ethics is required. Thus, the discomforting paradox of U.S. democracy becomes apparent: While we may desire a principle of equality that applies in exactly the same way to every citizen, in a society where equality is not guaranteed, we require historically sensitive principles that may appear to contradict the ideal of "equality." An historicized ethics operates toward the ideal of principles such as constitutional rights, but it also recognizes the need to develop ethical principles that take into account that not all persons have equal protection under the law or equal access to resources. Within a climate of extreme backlash to affirmative action and to women's rights, I propose an "affirmative action pedagogy," a pedagogy that ensures critical analysis within higher education classrooms of any expression of racism, homophobia, anti-Semitism, sexism, ableism, and classism. An affirmative action pedagogy seeks to ensure that we bear witness to marginalized voices in our classrooms, even at the minor cost of limiting dominant voices.

The first part of my argument is that all voices are not equal. Second, I will argue that the obligation of educators is not to guarantee a space that is free from hostility—an impossible and sanitizing task—but rather, to challenge oneself and one's students to critically analyze *any* statement made in a classroom, especially statements that are rooted in dominant ideological values that subordinate on the basis of race, gender, class, or sexual orientation. When students claim, for example, that they have been victimized by affirmative action, and "prove it" with their experience, we cannot allow ourselves or our students to be silenced by this "authority of experience" or "self-disclosure." No utterance that assumes the inferiority of targeted groups is sacred or immune to interrogation.

The Unique Public Spaces of Education

What does it mean to recognize, in the educational practices of college and university classrooms, that all voices are not equal? The solution is neither to invoke an absolutist sense of free speech, nor to prohibit simply and absolutely all hostile expressions. The uniqueness of classrooms is that, ideally, they provide a public space in which marginalized and silenced voices can respond to ignorant expressions rooted in privilege, white supremacy, or other dominant ideologies. Unlike many public spaces in which one may encounter hate speech—say, on a street or in a shopping mall—the classroom is one of the few public spaces in which one can respond and be heard. Educators must deal with messy issues that others cannot or do not want to address. Does this prerogative give educators any special constitutional privilege or dispensation? I leave that question open. However, to advocate that we use classrooms to critically interrogate racist and homophobic remarks is not based on an invocation of free speech. Rather, an affirmative action pedagogy recognizes that we are not equally protected in practice by the First Amendment, and that education needs to represent marginalized voices fairly by challenging dominant voices in the classroom.

I must also distinguish the public space of higher education classrooms from other public spaces where hate speech occurs. Within the majority of college and university classrooms, we are concerned with statements that are offensive, oppressive, or ignorant and that are supported by dominant cultural values institutionalized and validated through social, legal, and political practices. I distinguish such offensive expressions from what may be termed "verbal abuse" or what are legally referred to as "fighting words": for instance, name-calling solely intended to denigrate the other. [3]

The First Amendment protects the individual's right to free speech against government intervention. In the case of publicly funded higher education, the First Amendment protects individual educators' right to set classroom rules. However, to what extent does the First Amendment protect hostile expressions within classrooms? Within this murky legislative terrain, I set out to examine the ethics of affirmative action pedagogy. I want to explore a pedagogy that reflects a commitment as well to the Fourteenth Amendment and to Title IX, to ensure social equity and to create an educational climate that does not replicate the social inequities of the "real" world.

The Freedom to Create "Unreal" Spaces

Some argue that to create a classroom environment that does not replicate the inequities of the "real" world is a disservice to students. This accusation would apply as well to women's colleges and to historically black colleges. I can see no viable reason why educators should not create "separatist" spaces in which to empower historically marginalized groups, so that they may reenter a hostile "real" world better equipped to defend their views and rights. Universities in general function as "white men's clubs" and by default function to empower those who already hold privileged positions within the "real" world.

The highly publicized event, involving Professor Mary Daly's women's studies classroom has functioned as a lightning rod for these frequently ill-informed debates. Professor Daly made a decision to prohibit two male students from enrolling in her women's studies class. In this instance, apparently the two male students were enrolling not out of genuine educational interest but in a desire to "disrupt" the "safe space" of women's studies through contentious participation. I am told that Professor Daly regularly allowed men to enroll but held separate classes for them.

The Mary Daly case raises another interesting ethical dilemma: On what basis does one disallow a student from a classroom? In Daly's case, the intention of the prohibited students was precisely to disrupt the classroom environment. Yet in other cases, one may have students whose intention is not to disrupt, who are genuinely open to education and change, yet who bring with them potentially offensive views that can in effect disrupt the classroom as much as would intentional harassment.

Not all university educators, by any means, agree on what rules should govern the climate or speech of a classroom. At a recent women's studies faculty development meeting, we discussed how any of the 20 of us dealt with expressions of racist or homophobic ignorance that arise in our classrooms. One faculty member, an assistant professor in black studies, stated that she informs students that, during the semester, they are welcome to say or express any views they wish. She invites this precisely because she sees the classroom as a place where others can educate such ignorance, that collectively the group can respond and speak back. She described how she can see attitudes change within the context of the educational space, over time. For example, when she counters a student's ignorant remark, and other students chime in, she sees the student nodding his or her head as he or she begins to develop a new awareness of the social context of his or her expression. This professor stressed the importance of critical analysis: She requires students' accountability for every one of their claims and opinions.

Another assistant professor of religion and black studies expressed an entirely different set of ground rules. She described how her web page devotes a good portion to demarcating areas of discussion, questions, and remarks that are not permissible in her classroom. She discusses these rules of conduct with her students at the beginning of class. In a women's studies class, for example, she tells students that she expects that every enrolled student is there because he or she supports the empowerment of all women everywhere. In a black studies class, she tells enrolled students that she expects them to object to any denigration of black persons anywhere.

Is the second case an example of censorship? What if a student does not support the empowerment of women? However, what effects would it have if one excludes this student from class, when in fact there is some evidence to show that sitting through the course would change that person's prejudiced thinking? A program on PBS "Not in Our Town I" (Patrice O'Neill and Rhian Miller, directors, 1999) documented the radical transformation that can occur as a result of educational experience. Specifically, a course called "Tolerance" was offered in response to hate speech and crimes on a southern California high school campus. One semester a white supremacist attended the course but did not appear to change his views. A few years later, though, he returned to the teacher and explained how the course changed him. He reevaluated his belief system and now supports black rights.

Although the first instance—inviting students to express anything—may appear to invoke free speech, the operative principle is in fact, the belief that an educational environment actively engages critical analysis of how racist or homophobic opinions, for example, are founded in institutionalized systems of privilege and subordination. Following from this interpretation, the belief is that this process of challenging racism or homophobia will result in changing individual and group attitudes that are rooted in ignorance.

The second instance—prohibiting certain kinds of speech, or enforcing an assumption about what beliefs participants are assumed to hold—is similarly motivated by a commitment to an affirmative action pedagogy. In this type of classroom, it is significant that particular hostile expressions are prohibited—those aimed at subordinate groups. This rule functions to correct an educational history that has systematically discriminated against marginalized voices. Within women's and black studies in particular, this attempt to counter unequal representation is especially appropriate.

It is helpful to see both of the above pedagogies as different ways of deploying an affirmative action pedagogy. One encourages a voicing of the hostilities in order that they may be critically addressed; the other privileges marginalized voices by setting ground rules to create a space that allows, uniquely, the unheard to be heard.

Justifications for Historicized Ethics

On what basis might one justify an affirmative action pedagogy? The first justification is forwarded by legal scholars in the area of critical race theory. The authors of *Words That Wound* (Matsuda, Lawrence, Delgado, & Crenshaw, 1993) address the tension between the First and Fourteenth Amendment. The tension arises because, in fact, all people are not equally protected under the law because of the institutionalized inequities within our society. This reality complicates the effectiveness of the First Amendment. Scholarship in critical race theory and educational analyses document that in recent years, we find incidents of hate speech primarily to be directed at racial, religious, or sexual minorities. Not surprisingly, one finds in turn that invocations of the right to free speech are most often invocations to protect the right of the members of the dominant culture to express their hatred toward members of minority culture. These authors make important legal and historical cases to support their observation that, in practice, while the rhetoric of the First Amendment is a buzz word that makes all of us want to rally for its principle, in practice "the first amendment arms conscious and unconscious racists—Nazis and liberals alike—with a constitutional right to be racist. Racism is just another idea deserving of constitutional protection like all ideas" (Matsuda et al., 1993, p. 15). A scholar from another discipline addresses classroom dynamics and similarly argues that we must "read the appeal to the First Amendment as itself a kind of panic response in the same order as hate speech itself" (Roof, 1999, p. 45).

A second justification for privileging marginalized voices is based on the measurement of the psychological effect of hate speech on targeted groups and individuals. As one legal scholar explains, hate speech affects its victim in the visceral experience of a "disorienting powerlessness" (Lawrence, 1993, p. 70), an effect achieved because hate speech is comparable to an act of violence. In reaction to hate speech, the target commonly experiences a "state of semishock," nausea, and dizziness, and an inability to articulate a response. This scholar gives an example of a student who is white and gay. The student reports that in an instance where he was called "faggot" he experienced all of the above symptoms. However, when he was called "honky," he did not experience the disorienting powerlessness. As the scholar remarks, "the context of the power relationships in which the speech takes place, and the connection to violence must be considered as we decide how best to foster the freest and fullest dialogue within our communities" (Lawrence, 1993, p. 70).

These considerations bring me to another key point: The analysis of utterance in the classroom requires more than rational dialogue. In fact, the critical race theorists argue that because racism is irrational, no amount of rational dialogue will change racist attitudes. I disagree, in part because I am convinced that class-room discussion must recognize the emotions that shape and construct the meanings of our claims, our interchange with one another, and our investments in particular worldviews. Thus, a discussion of racism or homophobia cannot rely simply on rational exchange but must delve into the deeply emotional investments and associations that surround perceptions of difference and ideologies. One is potentially faced with allowing one's worldviews to be shattered, in itself a profoundly emotionally charged experience.

In her book *Excitable Speech*, Judith Butler makes an argument against the critical race theorists. Two aspects of her argument are relevant to mine: the accountability of the person who utters "hate speech," on the one hand, and the potential for critical agency on the part of the target of hate speech, on the other. Butler argues for the benefits of what she calls the "citationality of discourse which can work to enhance and intensify our sense of responsibility for it" (1997, p. 27). For example, the person who repeats or articulates a circulating form of hate speech should be required to negotiate "the legacies of usage that constrain and enable that speaker's speech" (1997, p. 27). Butler's argument reaches farther than my own, as she is arguing against any codes that constrain hate speech, including codes that might legislate hate speech in the dormitories or public spaces of a university. I am appropriating her point more narrowly to examine when and how injurious language expressed in a classroom provides a "teachable moment"—in other words, the extent to which educational spaces provide one of very few opportunities in which a speaker will be held accountable for the "legacies of usage" that surround offensive speech and beliefs.

I have frequently argued that one of the most effective ways to demand accountability for the "opinions" students feel "free" to express in the classroom, is a homework assignment that requires students to trace the source of their views. With respect to white supremacy, for example: a history of why and how it is condoned and supported, what enables the speaker as an individual to express this view without fear of censure or loss of privilege, and so forth. Such an assignment can be equivalently required of any student's expressed view: The sexual assault survivor can provide an analysis of the legacies that enable her to speak of being assaulted, of the histories of women's liberation that have sought to legislate on behalf of assault survivors, and so forth.

Butler's second point relevant to my discussion is her argument that the *expression* of hate speech, and not its censorship, is invaluable because such expressions ensure that the victims of hate speech can develop critical agency. She writes,

> Those who argue that hate-speech produces a "victim class" deny critical agency and tend to support an intervention in which agency is fully assumed by the state. In the place of state-sponsored censorship, a social and cultural struggle of language takes place in which agency is derived from injury, and injury countered through that very derivation. (1997, p. 41)

Butler's argument supports the black studies professor who invites her students to express any of their views, no matter how offensive. This argument is compelling in some educational situations, but it would seem to offer little in situations where there are no allies to the victim who risks his or her life in uttering a critical response. To tell someone who appears "gay" or "lesbian" that, when he or she is walking down the street and is accosted by homophobic remarks from a passing car that he or she should "engage in a social and cultural struggle over language" seems a rather empty promise of redress, given that there may be no opportunity to speak back or the person's life may be at risk. However, within an educational environment, articulation of injurious views can, if handled ethically, provide the target of hate speech with opportunities to speak back and thereby develop a sense of critical agency.

These complicating factors reiterate that all speech is not free and that the principle of free speech is so deeply mediated by power that it cannot assure the equality promised by democracy. I turn now to address briefly what has come to be called the "paradoxes of self-disclosure," which represent a post-political correctness use of "free speech" to protect hate speech.

"Self-Disclosure" as Thinly Disguised Hate Speech

Within a historical moment of backlash in which those with privilege have been "forced" by feminist and affirmative action policies to acknowledge power inequities, those with privilege have also recognized that expressions of "personal experience" tend to be exempted from penalization. An issue of *Concerns* (1999), a publication of the Modern Language Association, is devoted to the paradoxes created within the context of this backlash, particularly with respect to the First Amendment and new challenges for equitable pedagogies. The authors address an intriguing phenomenon of "self-disclosure" used by privileged students to justify offensive expressions. Self-disclosure essentially takes up where "non-situated" hate speech or assertions of superiority left off.

Judith Roof (1999) details the evolution of self-disclosure as a version of "standpoint epistemology," in which speakers locate themselves in relation to gender, race, class, and sexual orientation, for example. Roof goes on to argue that "the relative power accorded to groups in Western culture affects both what is disclosed and how that disclosure might be heard" (p. 48). As a result of differential weight and authority of voices,

> Self-disclosures sometimes manage, whether their tone is proud or apologetic, to validate the embattled attitudes of privilege and entitlement that tend to produce hate speech in the first place. Disclosure can transform a centrist or dominant position into a victimized, marginal, oppressed slot that competes loudly for attention against the more traditionally marginal and oppressed voices that are emerging . . . [resulting in] the reassertion of a speaker's relative privilege. (p. 49)

Many educators who teach about social inequalities encounter this phenomenon in which self-disclosure used by a speaker who enjoys relative social privilege functions to reassert their dominance. For philosophers, this throws us into longstanding arguments regarding epistemological relativism: Do all assertions carry equal weight? If not, why not? Particularly with respect to the invocation of "personal experience," how are we to "rank" the painfulness/attention-worthiness of different experiences, and how much space these experiences should be permitted within a discussion?

Angela Jones (1999) offers an insightful way of dealing with such uses of self-disclosure:

> Every semester, for instance, a self-identified white, middle-class male student will complain that he is tired of hearing minorities "whine" about their oppression, usually volunteering his own problems as evidence that he too is oppressed. . . . I resist the temptation to cross-examine him because his complaint typically shuts down anyone who would challenge him and my pointed questions would only shut him down or create an adversarial exchange. . . . Instead it is my goal at those moments to authorize those who have been silenced by connecting their previously volunteered experiences to this particular discussion. (p. 36)

The educator might then ask the marginalized students to discuss and explain the issues they have previously raised and bring the discussion around to ask: Why is it that analysis of racism and sexism gets cast as "whining"? Jones's example represents a recurrent problem: When we reconfigure the conversation to foreground the experiences of marginalized groups, those who have traditionally been at the center develop creative ways to reassert their centrality.

I recognize that my comment is contentious: Don't white, middle-class male students have as much right to share their experiences in the classroom? I think there are justifiable cases where they do not. In the case in question, the speaker's comment functions first to dismiss the other students' comments as "whining." Second, his interjection shifts the focus of attention back to himself and to his reluctance to recognize white male privilege as an institution and pervasive reality, no matter how troubled his own individual experience. If indeed the conversation then is redirected to his experience, affirmative action pedagogy fails. The discussion instead becomes one in which the privileged and dominant voice of society is the focus and center of attention, a context that further allows him to take up time justifying his emotional resistance to recognizing historically and socially determined inequities. Further, frequently such interjections derail a class from ongoing and in-depth study of nuances of feminist theory or other details of assigned readings. What is recreated is the classic situation to which women of color have learned to respond: "We don't want to educate you about racism, and we don't want to have to justify the fact of racism." This student's options include, instead, to go back over his class notes and assigned readings; discuss issues of sexism and feminism with other scholars and peers who care to educate him about sexism or racism, for example; to do further outside reading and scholarship to evaluate the extent of feminist, postcolonial, black, and cultural studies to grasp the accomplishments and breadth of cross-disciplinary critiques of privilege. Perhaps he can come to recognize that these critiques are not isolated instances of "whining" but rather part of a systematic investigation of social inequalities, hierarchies, and the operation of power within western society.

Putting Affirmative Action Pedagogy into Practice

The complexities of ensuring critical agency and juggling the paradoxes of self-disclosure come into sharp relief when one puts affirmative action pedagogy into practice. While I am arguing that ideally we challenge, for example, any homophobic remark uttered in a classroom, the complexity of social relations makes this extraordinarily difficult. To begin with, different voices carry different weight; some voices are heard better than others; some voices are foreclosed before even speaking. For example, it is one thing for my white male colleague to say, "As a heterosexual white man I believe that persons of any sexual orientation should be equally protected under the law." It is an entirely other matter for someone to say, "As a lesbian I believe that persons of any sexual orientation should be equally protected under the law." Obviously, the lesbian is biased while the white male heterosexual isn't, right? If the white man says "I feel victimized by affirmative action," the media and many of those in political power listen and validate his experience.

Whereas if an African American female says "I feel victimized by capitalist patriarchy" not only will she not be quoted in the news and not validated, she will be blamed for her failure to succeed.

A second level of complication surrounds the relationship between individuals, or between different group members. For example, I am thinking of a course I was co-teaching with an African American, heterosexual, female colleague. Early in the semester, the one African American male, who rarely said anything in class, stated, "I wouldn't want any homosexuals teaching my children." I experienced, to a degree, the visceral effects of hate speech. I was shocked by his comment. I was not out as a lesbian to this class. Frankly, at that particular moment, I didn't know how to respond. I also did not want to put this man on the spot, in part because he had not spoken before. I recall that my colleague spoke directly with him when we broke into small groups. In large part her ability to challenge him was founded in their shared racial identity and perhaps the fact of their shared sexual orientation.

I can recall in contrast an incident in another class in which the discussion was focused on issues of homophobia. A white male student shared, in a moment of self-disclosure, that the thought of two men having sex made him feel like throwing up, that it was totally disgusting and repulsive to him. He qualified by saying he was not opposed to other men being homosexuals, but—(the inevitable qualifier). In this instance, in part because I had established more of a sense of rapport and dialogue with this class and this young man, I was able to interrogate: "Why would one feel repulsion? What social institutions and values contribute to this being our learned response? Why, supposedly, don't we feel that when we think of heterosexuality?" These kinds of critical inquiry exemplify how teachers can demand accountability from students for their hostile expressions.

I want to briefly address further the experience of educators. Who can guarantee the safety of the educator? In my own experience, coming out at a public rally held on the drillfield of my university—a former military, engineering institution—in support of Matthew Shepherd was safer than coming out in my own classroom. In some ways for obvious reasons—because one assumed people attending a vigil for Shepherd support lesbian and gay rights; because I could slip away and never face that particular crowd again. However, it is a sad state of affairs that the fear of homophobia at this university is so great that many gay and lesbian professors and students I know do not come out. This means that gay and lesbian students in class have one less role model and ally.

Just as educators must commit to being allies to marginalized views within their classrooms, so must we develop creative ways to provide allies to the educator. Collaborative teaching with diverse instructors is an excellent way to create greater safety for an educator who feels silenced or fears recrimination from students or from the institution. For example, a woman defending feminism or addressing sexism will not always be heard as legitimate, whereas if a male colleague comes in and discusses feminism it lends validation. Crucially, for lesbian and gay educators who do not feel safe coming out it may be important to have straight allies come in and take some of the heat. This collaboration might be in the form of a roving "team" of colleagues who are available on an on-call basis. Although this is not an ideal solution—it risks disempowering the marginalized by requiring others to speak for them—it reiterates the fact that all speech is not free.

There are no prescriptions for one effective pedagogy. All speech is not equal, and this fact makes for a murky terrain with no easy solution. Ironically, one of the few places we may be able to exorcise some of the roots of inequality of speech is in the classroom, as painful and messy as this process may be. Until all voices are recognized equally, we must operate within a context of historicized ethics which consciously privileges the insurrectionary and dissenting voices, sometimes at the minor cost of silencing those voices that have been permitted dominant status for the past centuries.

Notes

1. Foreclosure is exemplified in the "Don't ask, Don't tell," policy applied to the presence of gays in the military.
2. See the many cases cited in Matsuda et al. For example, a 1989 case at Stanford University in which racist hate speech/vandalism was not penalized but a student of color protest faced disciplinary measures (1993, pp. 55–58).
3. This begs question of whether the simple utterance of a derogatory term, when invoked for the purpose of critical inquiry, is an instance of hate speech. See for example Butler (1997, pp. 37–40).

References

Butler, J. (1997). *Excitable speech*. New York: Routledge.

Jones, A. (1999). Self-disclosure in the feminist writing classroom. *Concerns: Publication of the Women's Caucus for the Modern Language Association, 26* (1), 33–41.

Matsuda, M., Lawrence, C., Delgado, R., & Crenshaw, K. (1993). *Words that wound*. Boulder: Westview Press.

Lawrence, C. (1993). If he hollers let him go: Regulating racist speech on campus. In M. Matsuda et al. *Words that wound* (pp. 68–81). Boulder: Westview Press.

Roof, J. (1999). The truth about disclosure, or revoking a First Amendment license to hate. *Concerns: Publication of the Women's Caucus for the Modern Language Association, 26* (1), 42–54.

Ronald David Glass

Moral and Political Clarity and Education as a Practice of Freedom

Classrooms that embody education as a practice of freedom cannot be made entirely safe. These learning environments are unavoidably risky in terms of the intellectual regions they engage, the emotional experiences they engender, the verbal exchanges they facilitate, and the actions they endorse. The volatile issues explored in them are among the most explosive and divisive in the culture, unearthing major fault lines that shake the foundations of meaning for individuals and society as a whole. Cognitive and emotional dissidence are necessary features of the critical consciousness and limit-acts that are among the objectives of liberatory courses. If the dominant ideologies are to be confronted and to some degree overcome, a variety of conflicts will be integral to this process. Discovering and articulating the realities underlying those ideologies, and questioning their effects within the identities and everyday practices of students, is often uncomfortable and even painful. Liberatory educators cannot promise a learning environment that protects everyone, and in fact, even after every precaution, they must themselves sometimes be the proximate cause of harms to students.

Thus, numerous moral and political issues emerge for liberatory educators in their classroom practices, and these are made even more urgent in the context of teacher education programs because the understandings and habits developed within them extend to impacts affecting countless numbers of children and youths. In addition, liberatory teacher educators face similar moral and political issues in relation to their faculty colleagues and the general climate of the colleges and universities. Proclamations of good intent cannot stop dominant ideologies from infecting even the most intimate recesses of learning environments from preschool through graduate school, and education as a practice of freedom entails constant vigilance, questioning, and challenging in the effort to make schools and universities positive forces in the struggle for justice and democracy.

This essay examines some moral and political dimensions of education as a practice of freedom in the context of confrontations with dominant ideologies as they manifest in the classrooms, hallways, offices, and meeting rooms of educational environments. In particular, it critiques certain misunderstandings of dialogue as it relates to those struggles and to liberatory classroom practices, and then articulates a more politically robust conception. This analysis lays the groundwork for an argument that moral and political clarity, not certainty, is required to understand the necessary actions and the obligatory relations entailed in these struggles, and also is required of every citizen actively engaged in the formation of a just democracy.

Dialogue, Limit-Situations, and Limit-Acts

Education cannot do everything, but still it can do something in the struggle for liberation (Freire, 1994, p. 91). Certain classrooms can be engines of liberation in unusual historical moments, such as during the late 1960s when university students in North America and Europe formed the leading edge of a global confrontation with the dominant military-industrial powers. Too often, however, the necessary linkage between these struggles and classrooms hoping to be liberating is overlooked. Paulo Freire, in his path setting *Pedagogy of the Oppressed* (1970/1994), developed a conception of education as a practice of freedom in which dialogue plays a central role. Many North American interpreters of Freire's theory mistakenly focused on dialogue as a method of conversation or discussion that could be applied in classrooms to make them liberating spaces (Aronowitz, 1993). They assumed that inclusion of student voices was necessarily empowering, and that a critical reading of oppressive features of reality was a cognitive achievement.

Freirean dialogue thus gets reduced to having students take turns speaking and insuring that each student participates, while the teacher avoids direct instruction for fear of reproducing oppressive relationships with the students. The misapprehension of the significance of discussion modalities is often linked to a similar conflation that occurs around content. Educators believe that reconstructing the curriculum to focus on counterhegemonic perspectives, discourses, and social realities will empower students, especially those represented within such perspectives, such as students of color and women. Once again, while these curricular transformations are important and offer some support for emancipatory projects, they alone, or in conjunction with a participatory approach to classroom discussion, can still easily miss the aim of education as a practice of freedom when they are not articulated to the struggles and limit-acts that secure freedom. This missed aim also clouds some of the recent discussion of ethical issues in classrooms hoping to contribute to counterhegemonic purposes.

The efforts of these teachers were certainly humanizing and a welcome advance over the predominant banking modes of education. However, they often amounted to a domestication of Freire's theory, overlooking the praxis that is essential to dialogue and the struggle for freedom (Glass, 2001a). Dialogue, when it is a liberatory praxis, is comprised of limit-acts that transcend, transform, or overcome limit-situations. Education as a practice of freedom is about conscious actions aimed at challenging ways of thinking and living that prevent people from realizing their own capacities for producing history, culture, and ways of life. A key to this praxis is the recognition of our situationality because it reveals "the very condition of existence" (Freire, 1970/1994, p. 90). In other words, it reveals the human power to make history and culture at the same time that historical and cultural realities shape human experience. People are submerged in realities that they have not necessarily consciously created with others, yet situations are not simply fated. They have specific concrete antecedents and always contain some recourse or room for free action within them. Critical reflection on the forces and entities that shape the situation uncover the obstacles, barriers, or boundaries (limit-situations) to that free action (self/class/group-defining/realizing action). Oppression is then overcome "by way of a breach with the real, concrete economic, political, social, ideological . . . order . . ." (Freire, 1994, p. 99). By getting some distance from experience, or emerging from our unconscious submersion within the dominant ideology, it is possible to uncover the *raison d'être* of the situation, recast its limits as problems open to transformative interventions, and identify "untested feasibilities" (realizable futures) beyond the present horizons that can be brought into being through struggle and effort.

Neither a critical knowledge of reality (especially socioeconomic structures and other major elements of the dominant ideology), nor language and speech that redefine that reality, are sufficient to change that reality without their being linked to the concrete struggle to transform the given situation. Frederick Douglass noted that "if there is no struggle, there is no progress" in regard to freedom and justice (Douglass, 1985, p. 204). It is crucially important that liberatory educators pay attention to the relationship between "political lucidity in a reading of the world, and the various levels of engagement in the process of mobilization and organization for the struggle for the defense of rights, for laying claim to justice" (Freire, 1994, p. 40). Dialogue, then, encompasses a wide array of methods that mediate the analysis of limit-situations and support the actions that comprise the struggle to transform that situation. Depending on the context and the political project at hand, lectures can be as emancipatory as a participatory discussion, and reactionary texts can be as illuminating and instrumental as revolutionary ones. What is crucial is moral and political clarity about the aims and methods so that the broader struggle for justice and democracy is served without moral and political inconsistency.

Dialogue and Silence

It should be clear by now that from the perspective of education as a practice of freedom, dialogue is not a conversation in which there is give and take among interlocutors in order to conduct an inquiry or debate, nor is it merely a pedagogical communicative relationship or a game played for the purpose of teaching and learning (Burbules, 1993). Teachers indeed employ dialogue in these various other forms, in the context of either conservative or progressive aims, and in addition, any or all of these conversational methods can be integrated to the dialogical praxis of education for liberation. In a similar vein, silence enfolds a range of meanings and significance that can embody contradictory political and pedagogical relationships, and that can vary by cultural contexts (Li, 2001). Silence can be a form of resistance to domination (and in this mode even be regarded as speech), and conversely it can be a manifestation of domination. The silence that is structured by economic, social, and political domination has been the particular concern of education as a practice of freedom, and in this context, a key transformative limit-act is the validation, empowerment, and amplification of the voices of the oppressed.

Some have raised questions about whether, for liberatory educators, a commitment to democratic dialogue also entails a commitment to tolerate voices in the classroom that give expression to the dominant ideology. This tolerance in effect resilences subaltern or counterhegemonic voices that have already been silenced by ideological structures imposed on the poor and working class, people of color, and women, for example. Thus, the question becomes whether an "affirmative action pedagogy" permits (and even requires) the silencing of these dominant voices/students (Boler, 2000). In assessing such questions, it must be kept in mind that these acts of silencing particular students or dominant ideologies in the classroom differ from one another in important moral and political ways, and, more pointedly, they have quite different substantive relationships with ideologically structured silence. Some of the force of this contrast can be brought out by analogy to the difference between a white person calling a black person "nigger" and a black person calling a white person "honky" or "cracker." While both insults are morally blameworthy, only the epithet "nigger" carries the force of a violent history of oppression that reinforces the threat and aggravates the harm done. Ideologically structured silence is pervasive, reinforced by a network of cultural practices and social institutions, and it maintains unjust economic, social, and political relations. Of course, the concern is precisely not to abet this structure of silence, allowing it to be reproduced in the liberatory classroom just at the moment when students disadvantaged by ideological silencing are being given space to find their voices.

The fact that the dominant voice in the classroom reinforces the structured silence of oppressive social conditions marks an important contrast to the silencing of that dominant voice. Even so, often only the silencing of the dominant voice is regarded as out of alignment with the democratic standards and norms of the society and of the supposedly fair equal opportunity of schools. The structural silencing of the poor, people of color, and women is not seen as such, and the pernicious effects of the dominant voice functions in an unspoken way within the background dynamics of the classroom. Either foregrounding these dynamics or silencing the dominant voice can then appear to uncritical eyes to be inconsistent with the articulated standards of democratic dialogue (all voices should be included) and also inconsistent with the formal and informal rules of classroom behavior of the educational institution. Students whose dominant voices are thus silenced may "get even" with faculty by assigning them unduly low scores on course evaluations, or by filing grievances that can lead to disciplinary action against those faculty. These threats can have chilling effects, especially on vulnerable faculty without tenure.

The moral and political differences associated with structural silences versus silencing particular students interconnect with others of significance in classrooms. Educators routinely silence certain voices and amplify others through the selection of the curriculum, the design of assignments and assessments, and the structure of the classroom social relations and learning environment. Each of these seeming pedagogical choices embeds ideological commitments that have real social, economic, and political consequences. Whereas the concrete content of these choices distinguish the liberatory from the reactionary or conservative educator/classroom to some degree, what most differentiates the liberatory educator/classroom is that these choices and actions are made subject to explicit critical examination rather than being left within hidden hegemonic practices. This includes making overt the moral and political commitments underlying the choices and shaping the intentions of study. In other words, the various forms of silencing that inhere within the dynamics of the classroom get identified as constituting elements of the limit-situation that require analysis and intervention in order to promote more just and more democratic educational and social institutions.

The political differences in these forms of silence and silencing have some bearing on the moral meaning and significance of the actions of the liberatory educator. The silences created in the structure of the class or by the individual educator's direct intervention in response to comments made by students cannot stand alone; the moral grounds of these choices must themselves be subject to critique. More specifically, the reasons for the choices must be given and analyzed. Neither moral nor political authoritarianism can be consistent with education as a practice of freedom. Silencing is not the problem, per se, but rather the issue is why and how it is achieved. After all, every dutiful parent at some moment silences a child in the child's own best interests or in order to meet the parental obligations to nurture, protect, and train the child, and so long as this is done nonviolently, selectively, and in ways supportive of the child's development, few would raise moral objections (Ruddick, 1989). Similar considerations bear on classrooms. Thus, even with sufficient grounds for some silencing in order to make space for nondominant perspectives, liberatory educators do not have license to silence students completely. Each student, regardless of his or her political views, is entitled to respect and to a voice within his or her educational experience. A liberatory educator in fact would want to insure that even the voice of the dominant has some place in the class if only to subject it to searching ideological critique. Perhaps it is thus better to think of the selective silencing of certain dominant discourses as a muting more than as a total elimination of that voice; and, after all, the dominant ideology blares from every corner of the culture, so there is no danger of it being utterly without expression even in a course in which each student embraced emancipatory politics and occupied a counterhegemonic identity position.

When it comes time to analyze the grounds for muting dominant voices and amplifying the voices of those silenced by the ideological structures of society, it is imperative that these actions not provide an excuse to hijack the agenda of the class. Often in these situations, students who embody dominant identity positions or who are committed to conservative political perspectives insist that the grounds for regulating discourse must satisfy their own criteria before they will agree to mute their voice and allow discussion to proceed along counterhegemonic lines. If, after thorough explanation and discussion, questions continue to be raised in good faith, these students can be provided with alternative means of extending their critique of the instructor's political and moral choices, such as by writing position papers or meeting with the instructor in an office hour outside class. Obstructive questioning must be clearly revealed as a tactical ploy aimed at reinforcing the same structure of silence that liberatory classes are attempting to subvert. Further, the instructor's authority can rightfully be exerted to prevent this obstruction to learning, just as with many other sorts of disruptive or threatening behavior that may occur in a classroom.

The muting of students cannot be dismissive of them or their learning and must occur within continuing moral, political, and pedagogical relationships and commitments. The tasks associated with these relationships and commitments constitute a portion of the struggle for justice within educational institutions and no doubt place substantive burdens on liberatory educators. However, education as a practice of freedom demands a sustained engagement with both ally and opponent in order to construct the kind of just and democratic community that animates dreams of a better future. Liberatory educators bear these burdens buoyed by moral and political clarity about the strategies and tactics of the struggle and their role within it. Their own lives must embody an ongoing effort at self-realization as they strive to demonstrate, however imperfectly, the modes of relation they hope for (hooks, 1994). Their own willingness to make these efforts transparent and subject to assessment announces a new context for teaching and learning that also supports the muting, criticism, and denunciations that are a necessary part of the struggle for justice. While any pedagogical approach results in some harms to some students, these are left unexamined except in education as a practice of freedom, where public reflection and deliberation locate them within larger moral and political frames.

Moral Clarity, Struggle, and Dirty Hands

Few people, whether conservative or progressive, will acknowledge the ways in which they manifest dominant ideologies, and even fewer graciously accept being criticized for it. Even so, it is impossible for anyone born into and raised within our society not to in some degree inhabit, and be inhabited by, the dominant ideologies (Glass, 2000). Racism, sexism, classism, linguicism, and ability-ism each mark our habits of mind and body, infusing the most intimate and sacred just as surely as the most public and profane. Thus, liberatory educators cannot claim some position of righteousness in regard to the dominant ideologies of the day any more than they can claim a kind of perfection that escapes the ordinary vices that preoccupy most everyday moral discourse (Shklar, 1984). In fact, even to aspire to a moral purity that is beyond racism, sexism, and so forth, is to hope for the wrong thing. The best one can hope for is to become more effective and committed in the struggle against racism, sexism, classism, and so on, and in the struggle for justice and democracy. Moral clarity enables teachers and learners to grasp that each of us is inextricably implicated in both what we struggle against and what we struggle for, and thus to criticize others with more understanding and compassion, and with a greater capacity to engage them in their own ongoing quest for moral betterment. Humility is thus not an attribute of a saint or of a sinner, but rather it should be a consequence of political insight into the structure of oppression, the processes of ideological formation, and the challenges of realizing justice and democracy. The degree to which any of us is innocent is often more a matter of moral luck than it is a matter of discreet choices (Williams, 1981), and even in the most extreme situations of violence and oppression, such as the Nazi concentration camps, a moral gray zone predominates over stark contrasts of good and evil, right and wrong (Levi, 1988).

Persistent moral ambiguities and inescapable moral and political contradictions within both society and individual lives thus entail cautious judgments. Competing moral conceptions and their diverse goods, aims, and judgments contribute additional weight to such caution. This diversity is found not only across cultural differences that span the globe, but also within the pluralistic dynamics of western societies, and even more so among those aspiring to democratic and just arrangements. In fact, there is good reason to regard moralities as akin to natural languages, defying easy or certain translation from one to another, and without the possibility of an ultimate arbiter among them or the ways of life tied to each (Hampshire, 1983).

Caution need not become paralysis, with judgment confined to a despairing nihilism that either denies the possibility of any substantive moral grounding or asserts the moral equivalence of all views or actions. Moral clarity is not moral certainty, but it still carries sufficient force to overcome relativistic positions and orient liberatory practices that criticize or condemn oppression's surface appearances and deep structures. "Of course, the element of punishment, penalty, correction—the punitive element in the struggle we wage in our hope, in our conviction of its ethical and historical rightness—belongs to the pedagogical nature of the political process of which struggle is an expression" (Freire, 1994, p. 9). If justice is to mean anything at all, it must be made concrete in relation to specific abuses and injustices that are named as such and corrected or overcome on the basis of consistent and explicit principles and rationales. Tolerance and empathy for people who manifest dominant ideologies or who oppose a critical reading of the world do not require passivity. In addition, moral and caring relationships do not supercede the need for a radical commitment to the political struggle that challenges those ideologies and the unjust privileges conferred on some while disadvantages are heaped on others. Liberatory classrooms can never be neutral, and by facilitating searching investigations of the ideological formations inhabiting common sense and the habitual ways of being of everyone in schools and colleges, they "comfort the afflicted and afflict the comfortable" in the effort to build democratic movements for justice. Civility blocks needed critiques and can be a barrier to change since the underlying structures of good manners themselves favor the powerful (Mayo, 2001, 2002). To call attention to the underlying dominant ideologies gets labeled as provocative by those who benefit from the silence (Thompson, 2001). However, just such provocations are necessary to open transformative possibilities within situations.

Without a settled account of a universal moral calculus, moral and political conflicts will be endemic to a pluralistic society, placing a premium on rules of procedural justice that minimally insure free speech and the opportunity to make a case for particular conceptions of the good (Hampshire, 1983). In fact, established mechanisms for nonviolently handling such disagreements through deliberative processes are precisely what distinguish healthy democracies from other forms of political arrangements (Gutmann & Thompson, 1996). Thus, a capacity for active participation in these moral and political conflicts and deliberations is both central to democratic citizenship and to the aims of education as a practice of freedom. These conflicts and deliberations can be decidedly messy. Therefore, liberatory educators' moral and political clarity about these dynamics must undergird their denunciations of dominant ideologies and insure their efforts to make judgments transparent and open to criticism. Nonetheless, because education as a practice of freedom entails direct action to challenge dominant ideologies and to support the formation of more just and democratic institutions, the moral dilemmas in these struggles are not merely matters of debate and discussion. When we make certain choices and act in accord with them, positive harms can befall those who are not precisely blameworthy.

For example, through no fault of their own, students embody and proclaim dominant ideologies that have inhabited them unawares. When liberatory educators silence or correct these students, even though for a good cause and with care, the students may experience this negatively. Those students' sense of efficacy or moral agency or their stature with other students may be diminished, at least temporarily. More generally, all students in the class may be harmed to some degree if a seeming display of ends justifying inconsistent means reinforces a sense of moral cynicism. These moral harms are certainly relatively minor and have limited social, economic, and political scope when compared with the ill effects resulting from other educational and political decisions or from the outcomes and logics of the dominant ideologies. Nonetheless, the transgressions that produce harms in the course of education as a practice of freedom dirty the hands of liberatory educators and carry their own particular burdens (Glass, 2001b). When action is taken in the broader public arenas of power and politics, negative effects grow commensurately more serious. For those who struggle for justice and democracy, innocence has no place.

Some have hoped that the moral burdens that come with the dirty hands acquired in striking blows against injustices and dominant ideologies are to some degree cleansed by duties that command stronger allegiance and justify transgressions against individuals. It might be argued that liberatory educators are acting toward paramount goals that serve the common good, and that they have a professional responsibility to make decisions about the curriculum and its implementation and to shape the behavior of students through coercive measures that assess and grade their performance. If students are harmed as a secondary "double effect" of such actions after due precautions, then no moral blame accrues to the educator, whose conscience can be clear. This reasoning seems to absolve blame by means of a utilitarian discounting of the harms done to some students, whereas other approaches achieve the same effect by other routes. For example, realists in the Machiavellian tradition argue that decisions lack substantive moral content when taken within situations amenable only to calculations of utility, and therefore they should be judged solely by practical results and not morally. In such cases, they argue, moral considerations apply only to the character of the person making the choices or exercising power. In other words, it is necessary to make sure that the educator has reliable moral habits and inflicts harm only as necessary to secure the best possible lives for all the students taken together. In this view, individual students harmed once again have no special claim on the conscience of the educator.

These justifications of harms done while advancing the cause of justice in liberatory classrooms—whether by way of universal principles in line with the highest duties, or of a utilitarian calculus seeking the greatest good, or of the amoral pragmatics of the realist—share an assumption that accepts a split between public and private virtue. That is, these views hold that otherwise good people who are the proximate cause of harms done to innocents bear no moral burdens for those actions so long as they acted conscientiously, and thus their personal virtue remains unsullied by their public sin. Some have sought to mend this rift between public and private virtue by suggesting two alternative outlooks (see Walzer, 1974). One perspective is that good people who commit harms in order to do good should be anguished by their choices and transgressions, and suffer from understanding that neither worthy reasons nor beneficial results can prevent a tragic "loss of soul" as their fate. In this case, repentance salves the soul without fully healing it or restoring lost innocence, so the agony of this loss is deepened by recognition of its permanence. This moral tragedy remains largely private, although a second, more heroic, possibility is available. In this latter case, private anguish is augmented by public acknowledgment of the wrong done and acceptance of judgment and perhaps even punishment. Whereas these moral psychologies provide greater consistency in coping with the problem of dirty hands, they still fall short of the radical commitments necessary for education as a practice of freedom (Glass, 2001b).

At the same time that education as a practice of freedom recognizes that perfection is impossible, it requires neither tragic suffering nor heroism. In the context of multiple conceptions of the good, each with distinctive ways of life adhering to a diversity of competing principles and methods of moral calculation, it does not seek moral certainty. Rather, education as a practice of freedom seeks to create conditions that reveal both public and private moral life as continually negotiated compromises and that support the formation of citizens actively involved in those negotiations. Such citizens are also committed to struggle for justice and democracy against the weight of ideological forces that skew moral deliberations. Liberatory actions in classrooms and society do not have the luxury of having their associated moral burdens washed away by rationalized justifications. Instead they are grounded within genuine moral dilemmas that result in harm to innocents. All educators inevitably mute or silence some while amplifying and giving voice to others in line with their moral, political, and educational choices. Liberatory educators try to make their choices in favor of justice, democracy, and the oppressed, and in opposition to inequity and dominant ideologies. Such choices cannot avoid harm one way or another, and because those harmed have moral standing as persons regardless of their views or behaviors, liberatory educators are challenged to recognize them and give their experience its own measure of moral weight. The dilemmas of political and moral action leave unfinished remainders (see Gowans, 1987) that obligate liberatory educators to remain connected with allies and opponents alike in the ongoing deliberations, negotiations, and struggles that literally comprise moral and political life within pluralistic democracies.

Moral and political clarity is the understanding of these dilemmas and obligations, which provides a strategic foundation for actions that challenge the situational limits that prevent every person from fulfilling their human capacity to make history and culture. Within the struggle to build the just, democratic society necessary to insure that this capacity is concretely realized for everyone, liberatory educators try to construct transformative relationships with those students, faculty, and staff with whom they agree and are in political solidarity, but also those with whom they disagree or with whom they are in conflict. The precariousness of the dominant ideology (despite its bedrock power) and the persistent possibility of the conversion of opponents to the cause of justice are features of every situation, and they sustain a radical hope and militancy. To truly transform oppressive ways of life and the people and institutions that animate and support them, liberatory educators and their allies have no other consistent strategic choice but to remain in relation with the dominant classes and institutions that are enemies of justice and democracy so as to understand and challenge them. These relationships are certainly very difficult, emotionally and politically. They are a kind of spiritual task taken on in light of a clear understanding of the difficulty of making present a more just and democratic future. This approach to liberatory education reinvents power without moral righteousness about the certainty of the best path to reach the dream that draws us forward. There is no finish to such work; the struggle for a just democracy is a way of life, that of the citizen.

Struggle and Citizenship

Students coming from and heading toward all walks of life need to understand their "own selves as historical, political, social, cultural beings" and in doing so thus comprehend "how society works" (Freire, 1994, p. 133). This "route to the invention of citizenship" (Freire, 1994, p. 39) cannot be taken through training, but rather must be achieved by education that embodies the ongoing critique of reality, empowers the voices, hopes, and aims of formerly silenced groups, and encourages systematic conjectures toward and anticipations of justice and democracy. To become strong and active citizens able to resist the dominant ideology and build a more just and democratic future, students must be enabled to overcome the "existential weariness" and "historical anesthesia" that undermines their efficacy and keeps them immersed in "personal problems and concerns of the moment, unable to glimpse the 'untested feasibility' that lies beyond the 'limit-situation'" (Freire, 1994, p. 137). When students discern the boundaries of their existence and their transcending power to make history and culture, they can engage the struggle for the future strategically and responsibly.

In a liberatory classroom, as students come to understand how oppression and the dominant ideologies shape their lives (whether they enjoy the privileges or suffer the consequences of that dominant order), oppression passes from being simply a weight to bear to becoming an opportunity, a challenge, a situation calling for creative insight and response. A classroom committed to collaborative ongoing criticism of the totality of life uncovers the dynamics of culture and history, revealing the given situation or what has come down through tradition as processes in which everyone continues to play a role. That role is subject to some personal and collective control, so the dominant ideology can be countered, blocked, and resisted, while at the same time new meanings and ways of being are constructed, drawing on the struggles of the past to build up already present possibilities. Liberatory classrooms must facilitate students' actual lived production of a more just and democratic society, "created, politically produced, worked on, in the sweat of one's brow, in concrete history" (Freire, 1994, p. 157).

In other words, education as a practice of freedom links learning to the "political process of the battle for citizenship" (Freire, 1994, p. 199). It establishes forms of ethics and politics that will not defeat justice and democracy on the way toward their realization. The directive and political nature of this education accentuates a need for an ethics of respect geared into the fight for justice. Respect for differences and for those who oppose the liberation of the oppressed can be maintained even as liberatory educators testify for and defend their political choices and challenge the limiting conditions of their situation. We can respect opponents who reinforce the dominant ideologies, even as we combat their positions and powers "earnestly and with passion" (Freire, 1994, p. 79).

Given present historical circumstances, the direct engagement in the struggle against dominant ideologies and in the construction of a more democratic and just society inevitably leads citizens to violate state laws and public conventional standards in order to serve moral and political interests. Education as a practice of freedom consequently requires preparation for the transgressions integral to active citizenship. In order to overcome the structures, standards, and forms of power articulated with institutionalized dominant ideologies, yet without reproducing those ideologies and modes of relation (merely replacing the old oppressor with the formerly oppressed), it is best if liberation struggles practice militant nonviolence (Glass, 1996). This strategic approach to social change has animated twentieth-century campaigns in countries that span the globe and includes confrontations with regimes backed by some of the largest armies in the world (Powers & Vogele, 1997; Zunes, Kurtz, & Asher, 1997). The limit-acts that challenge injustice and still embody principles of respect, care, and justice can be developed along a strategic continuum; moral considerations need not disable forceful political action (King, 1963). From myriad forms of noncooperation with injustice that open the struggle to participation, even by children, to more confrontational tactics that include strikes, boycotts, and direct actions that prevent business as usual, militant nonviolence offers an array of options to counter dominant ideologies, to build democratic institutions, and to provide for national security (Sharp, 1973, 1985).

Given the inequities and injustices of the day as reflected in dominant ideologies such as racism, sexism, classism, linguicism, and ability-ism, education as a practice of freedom must foster the capacity to participate in militant nonviolent campaigns. Civil disobedience that challenges governmental authority can be expected as part of the healthy functioning of democratic and nearly just societies (Rawls, 1971). In fact, this capacity for struggle should be regarded as one of the foundational skills of citizenship. However, citizens who embody these practices cannot wrap themselves in flags of righteousness or be armored with moral certainty. Even with right on the side of overcoming oppression and promoting just, democratic ways of life, these struggles cannot lay claim to infallible knowledge and understanding and cannot avoid at least some harm to innocents. Dirty hands come with conscientious citizenship. Therefore, education as a practice of freedom must do more than hone moral sensibilities and reason and more than heighten commitment to moral action. Citizenship in the service of justice and democracy requires the open bearing of moral burdens coupled with unrelenting struggle to create a future now only imagined.

Alone among strategies for the radical transformation of unjust societies, militant nonviolence embraces the uncertainties and varieties of reason in knowledge, respects the plural compelling conceptions of the good that can shape democracy, and recognizes the malleability and contradictions of identity (Glass, 2000). The cultural and historical praxis that is at the heart of human existence provides the "opportunity of setting ourselves free" insofar as we join the "political struggle for transformation of the world" (Freire, 1994, p. 100). When this political and ideological fight is wedded to militant nonviolence, it becomes a strategy that makes more credible the demand that citizenship entail a permanent radical struggle for justice and democracy because it preserves to all equally the power to seek self-determined hopes and dreams. Education as a practice of freedom both engenders and draws upon this understanding of citizenship. It gears itself into these struggles and makes sure that schools and classrooms that pursue it become sites of personal and social change, and contribute to the embodiment of greater justice and democracy.

Classroom Practices

Perhaps a brief discussion of my own current classroom practices can illuminate the meaning of linking education as a practice of freedom with the formation of citizens committed to the struggle for justice and democracy. I, like most faculty members in colleges of education, teach far from the front lines and under the gaze of unsympathetic authorities. In my university, students are primarily working-class white adults who are the first members of their families to be obtaining a university degree. For the most part, they reflect the rightist political ideologies of the state's long-ruling Republican party and the evangelical conservative Christian theology of the dominant local religions. If my courses were not required for graduation with bachelor's or master's degrees in education, it would be safe to bet that enrollment would be a tiny fraction of what it is. In this context, it is liberating merely to crack the certainty of the meanings that define their everyday world and self-understandings while, at the same time, enabling their sense of wonder about and engagement with the issues at hand. Nonetheless, I expect more, despite the fact that these required core courses cannot be structured strictly in alignment with the principles of education as a practice of freedom due to institutional constraints.

My "ground rules" for discussion and interaction point immediately toward a transformative agenda: the importance of separating views from persons and an insistence on respect for all persons; a recognition that ideological purity or complete goodness are impossible, and that every student and teacher, regardless of how long they have struggled against the dominant ideologies, is still shaped and infected by those ideologies; a commitment not to focus on blame but rather to take responsibility for the reality and limit-situations investigated in the class; a willingness to examine issues deeply, following ideological traces into hidden or obscure areas of both public and private life; an understanding of the uncertainties of interpreting ideological markers in situations, and a commitment to the rigors of study and modes of investigation that warrant knowledge; and, an openness to taking actions that can lead to transforming one's self and the situation. I do not expect students to agree with me, or with each other, but I do expect them to be moved in some profound way by what we discover and do together in the process of investigating the course topics. I explicitly tell students on the first day of class that insofar as they participate fully in the class, they will never be the same. This substantive objective may seem grandiose for a mere 45 hours or less of class time, but it puts students on notice about the difficult and sometimes scary process ahead, and it begins to open up the possibility of irrevocable change.

I use an assortment of readings and films that contain autobiographical accounts of ordinary people grappling with dominant ideologies, thus challenging students to think about what they might do with their own lives. In class discussions and written assignments, I pose questions that defy set or easy answers, that uncover hidden structures behind surface appearances, and that provoke uncertainty in students' understandings of what they take for granted. To foster this critical reading of the world, popular culture can often provide a starting place to reveal the underlying contradictions within their identities and their world. I encourage multiple, even antagonistic, interpretations and analyses in order to disclose the ideological forces at work in constructing everyday experience. I steadfastly oppose dogmatism and certainties, and instead encourage and support students' curiosity so that they can become active investigators of themselves and their reality, always engaged in an ongoing quest for the "why?" of the world.

Saul Alinsky famously remarked that effective community organizers had to "rub raw the resentments of the people of the community" (Alinsky, 1989, p. 116). In other words, he knew that the wounds inflicted by injustice produced injuries that could not be healed without first opening them up and then cleaning them so healing could begin. I, too, expose the sore points in the culture, knowing that without an explicit recognition that many people are suffering from the current political, social, economic, and cultural orders, people will be little likely to undertake the additional suffering required to transform that reality. I acknowledge the pain that comes with recognition of one's ignorance and implicit contribution to evil, and identify these experiences in my own life. I widen the breach with the everyday commonsense understandings of self and society that leave students feeling vulnerable, because these breaches and vulnerabilities are needed for them to see reality more clearly. By fostering the strangeness that emerges with the first glimmerings of critical insight, I provoke significant anxiety and cause tensions in students' close relationships. However, only in the space of this strangeness and anxious tension can an understanding develop of the mechanisms and forces that produce reality and of the new possibilities that fill the situation. Only by helping students pass through this sense of alienation from who they were and what they knew before, can I assist them to free their imaginations to see how things might be otherwise. By providing detailed examples of movements that have transformed the society they now take as a given, I encourage students to grasp the actions within their own reach that can bring the future into the present. In their efforts to embody this new reality, they learn that the changes must be forged in the crucible of struggle.

The hard, even grueling, work entailed in these courses imposes a special obligation on me to make myself extraordinarily available for office hours to support students as they wrestle with the challenges of becoming more consistent with their intentions and dreams. The revelation of reality is not necessarily motivation to transform reality. Not only do the fear of freedom and the outright denial of ordinary people's power to make history and culture block a critical understanding of the dynamics of self-class-race-gender-reality formation, they also block an ability to commit to the struggle. Additional psychological factors bear on the fruitfulness of courses based on education as a practice of freedom, and these are often best addressed one-on-one in extended office hours. The truth of oppression and the power of the dominant ideology in our lives can be humiliating and reinforce a sense of incompetence, fostering even overwhelming feelings of guilt and shame at being thus dominated or controlled by forces beyond us. These feelings of humiliation, guilt, shame, and weakness must themselves become objects of critical reflection and be linked to the reality that must be denounced and actively resisted. At the same time, students' personal histories must be linked to the long public history of struggle and sacrifice inherited from an ongoing community of freedom fighters to which students can become connected. As they begin to understand critically the mechanisms of social conflict, they can participate in their own way in the ongoing battles that mark their age and generation.

Beyond the classroom, I make my own life an example of commitment to the tasks necessary to transform the climate and structures of the college, university, and community. I build community and leadership through organizing social activities as well as political actions, through networking and connecting like-minded people, and through mentoring young talented students and supporting them into significant volunteer and employment opportunities. I engage in almost daily resistance activities that press themselves into my schedule regardless of how burdened I may be. These are things that give no choice about time and place for action, but require immediate response. The force of the dominant ideology assaults vulnerable people in small and large ways, and given that I enjoy the benefits of race, class, and gender privileges, it is especially incumbent on me to intervene in a wide variety of both public and private ways as necessary to protect people and principles. I take public stands on the issues of the day, even if only to reiterate principles of justice in the face of defeat, or to refuse cooperation with policies or actions that are affronts to fairness. I attend meetings, serve on committees, write letters, make phone calls, sign petitions, and monitor the actions of opponents. As I have aged and to some degree grown wiser, I have gained greater effectiveness by balancing my relentless practice of resistance and critique with similarly everyday practices that embody justice and democracy. Often these practices take the personal form of spiritual work to reduce my negativity and cynicism, to increase my kindness and compassion, to be more forgiving, and to be more mindful of my family. In addition, I try to embody the changes I seek by joining with others who are like-minded in organizations and communities that are actively making a difference. By trying my best, not deterred by always falling short, I hope to demonstrate another way to lead a life that takes citizenship seriously and struggles toward the realization of the just democracy that is our nation's promise.

Concluding Comments

It is easy to slip into despair in the face of the tremendous challenges that inhibit the realization of a just democracy. Each of us individually can seem so small in comparison to the size of the task. The relentless press of the dominant ideologies leaves no space for respite. The burdens of liberatory work weigh on our emotions and sap our energy. The temptations to forget the struggle and lose oneself in the oblivions of consumerism and escapism flood the mass media. The righteous demands and needs of our loved ones and friends are sufficient to occupy us without the added responsibilities of repairing the world. The calls to study other important matters pervade schools and colleges, and assessments that foretell our future opportunities pay scant attention to the issues of justice and democracy.

Each of us must first realize that just as we are not responsible for the entire task of liberation, of building a just democratic society, so we are nonetheless obligated to do something. When our aim is large, no task is too small. When so much is to be done, every effort makes some contribution. As more and more people take up the challenge to press the limits of their particular situations, and as these efforts are linked in broader struggle, the wheel of history can be turned to realize the ancient dream of justice for all. Few callings, if any, are higher than to be a citizen who forces such movement, and few aims, if any, are as worthy of directing education.

Note

This essay was substantively improved by comments on an earlier draft that were provided by Pia Lindquist Wong; all remaining deficiencies and obscurities remain my sole responsibility. Portions of this essay in the section entitled "Moral Clarity, Struggle and Dirty Hands" draw from an earlier work: On transgression, Moral Education, and Education as a Practice of Freedom, *Philosophy of Education 2001* [S. Rice (Ed.), Urbana, IL: Philosophy of Education Society, University of Illinois at Urbana-Champaign], pp. 120–128.

References

Alinsky, S. D. (1989). *Rules for radicals.* New York: Vintage Books.

Aronowitz, S. (1993). Paulo Freire's radical democratic humanism. In P. McLaren & P. Leonard (Eds.), *Paulo Freire: A critical encounter* (pp. 8–24). New York: Routledge.

Boler, M. (2000). All speech is not free: The ethics of "affirmative action pedagogy." In L. Stone (Ed.), *Philosophy of education 2000* (pp. 321–329). Urbana, IL: Philosophy of Education. Society, University of Illinois at Urbana-Champaign.

Burbules, N. C. (1993). *Dialogue in teaching.* New York: Teachers College Press.

Douglass, F. (1985). In J. W. Blassingame (Ed.), *The Frederick Douglass papers. Series 1: Speeches, debates, and interviews. Vol. 3: 1855–63.* New Haven: Yale University Press.

Freire, P. (1994a). *Pedagogy of hope.* New York: Continuum.

Freire, P. (1994b). *Pedagogy of the oppressed.* New York: Continuum. (Original work published in 1970).

Glass, R. D. (1996). *On Paulo Freire's theory of liberation education, and nonviolence.* Stanford University, Stanford, CA.

Glass, R. D. (2000). Education and the ethics of democratic citizenship. *Studies in Philosophy and Education, 19*(3), 275–296.

Glass, R. D. (2001a). On transgression, moral education, and education as a practice of freedom. In S. Rice (Ed.), *Philosophy of education 2001* (pp. 120–128). Urbana, IL: Philosophy of Education Society, University of Illinois at Urbana-Champaign.

Glass, R. D. (2001b). Paulo Freire's philosophy of praxis and the foundations of liberation education. *Educational Researcher, 30*(2), 15–25.

Gowans, C. W. (1987). *Moral dilemmas.* New York: Oxford University Press.

Gutmann, A., & Thompson, D. (1996). *Democracy and disagreement.* Cambridge: The Belknap Press of Harvard University Press.

Hampshire, S. (1983). *Morality and conflict.* Cambridge: Harvard University Press.

hooks, b. (1994). *Teaching to transgress: Education as the practice of freedom.* New York: Routledge.

King, M. L., Jr. (1963). Letter from a Birmingham Jail. In *Why we can't wait* (pp. 77–100). New York: Harper and Row.

Levi, P. (1988). *The drowned and the saved* (R. Rosenthal, Trans.). New York: Summit Books of Simon & Schuster, Inc.

Li, H.-L. (2001). Silences and silencing silences. In S. Rice (Ed.), *Philosophy of Education 2001* (pp. 157–165). Urbana, IL: Philosophy of Education Society, University of Illinois at Urbana-Champaign.

Mayo, C. (2001). Civility and its discontents: Sexuality, race, and the lure of beautiful manners. In S. Rice (Ed.), *Philosophy of Education 2001* (pp. 78–87). Urbana, IL: Philosophy of Education Society, University of Illinois at Urbana-Champaign.

Mayo, C. (2002). The ties that bind: Civility and social difference. *Educational Theory, 52*(2), 169–186.

Powers, R. S., & Vogele, W. B. (Eds.). (1997). *Protest, power, and change: An encyclopedia of nonviolent action from ACT-UP to women's suffrage.* New York: Garland.

Rawls, J. (1971). *A theory of justice.* Cambridge: The Belknap Press of Harvard University Press.

Ruddick, S. (1989). *Maternal thinking: Toward a politics of peace.* Boston: Beacon Press.

Sharp, G. (1973). *The politics of nonviolent action.* Boston: Porter Sargent.

Sharp, G. (1985). *National security through civilian-based defense.* Omaha, NE: Association for Transarmament Studies.

Shklar, J. N. (1984). *Ordinary vices.* Cambridge: The Belknap Press of Harvard University Press.

Thompson, A. (2001). Agent provocateuse. In S. Rice (Ed.), *Philosophy of education 2001* (pp. 88–91). Urbana, IL: Philosophy of Education Society, University of Illinois at Urbana-Champaign.

Walzer, M. (1974). Political action: The problem of dirty hands. In M. Cohen, T. Nagel & T. Scanlon (Eds.), *War and moral responsibility* (pp. 62–84). Princeton, NJ: Princeton University Press.

Williams, B. (1981). *Moral luck: Philosophical papers 1973–1980.* Cambridge: Cambridge University Press.

Zunes, S., Kutz, L. R., & Asher, S. B. (Eds.). (1999). *Nonviolent social movements: A geographical perspective.* Oxford: Blackwell.

Cris Mayo

The Tolerance That Dare Not Speak Its Name

Recently I have been asking queer college students to recall their public school experiences. I have received a pattern of oddly contradictory responses that turn out not to be contradictions at all. I ask, "Have you ever experienced harassment of any kind because you were queer?" Many of the respondents begin their answers with something like "No, I didn't experience harassment, what happened was no big deal, nothing out of the ordinary." They then, having framed their experience as ordinary, recount harassment from teachers and students, harassment from students in front of teachers who did nothing, and physical harassment. Surprisingly, though they emphasize that they expected that kind of behavior, and even if, on further reconsideration, they acknowledge that it is unacceptable, they understand it to have been normal and unremarkable. As one young man put it, "No one really frowned upon it [homosexuality], but no one talked about it." He then said he remembered "maybe one bad thing." It turned out that he had had his head smashed into a locker because other students thought he was gay, but he said "I felt it wasn't that bad of an action." In addition to what other students did to them, respondents point out the official silence, the lack of information, and the lack of teacher and administrator attention to the homophobic speech and action. All their schools, of course, had policies intent on protecting students from harassment. However, none of the schools had policies that specifically protected sexual minority students. Thus, part of the problem was that the kind of speech that harassed sexual minority students was not understood by the school community to be harassment. Homophobic speech was just what queer kids should expect. I contend in this paper that because the structure of social institutions and practices fuels homophobia, that even with policies to protect them, homophobia is still what queer people can expect. Even policies and rules that purport to protect sexual minority students will not work because they are still guided by institutions intent on maintaining a veneer of acceptance of sexual minorities through the establishment of conduct codes centralizing individual agency. Though individual acts are sanctioned, schools as institutions continue to engage in substantially discriminatory practices.

The policies that I examine in this paper are indicative of the intentional shortsightedness that maintains dominance while appearing to protect sexual minority students, as well as other students, in public schools. I will argue that policies are written to prevent substantive change by focusing on simple, reactive rules rather than large-scale changes in curricula or social practices. To examine how adding rules is meant to limit larger changes, I analyze nondiscrimination policies in Massachusetts and Maryland that curtail curricular representation of sexual minority issues. I then turn to an examination of the decision in *Saxe v. State College Area School District* that cancelled a broadly protective speech code in Pennsylvania. In each of these cases I will show that policies are more intent on regulating speakers of words than encouraging learning and community. Rules and rulings about rules continue the intentional silencing and trivializing of sexual minority students. Even the anti-homophobia demonstration most popular in public schools, "Day of Silence" requires silencing. While the intentional silence required by the "Day of Silence" does pose some difficulties for imagining what a vibrant community of sexual diversity would look like, I will argue that the intentional self-silencing draws productive attention to the unproductive silences policies attempt to enforce.

Civil Speech and Curricular Silence

While the damage done by hateful speech is considerable, we need to think more broadly about the context in which that speech takes place as well as the tendency for codes of conduct to focus on individual action. While it may be tempting to say that all laws and rules ultimately require that individuals control themselves for the good of the community, laws and rules also cover over the situation in which individuals act. The particular acts of harassment that occur in public schools are so damaging because they occur in contexts that are pervasively homophobic, not only because of individual action but institutional arrangement. Schools do not address issues of concern to sexual minority students or to students at all curious about sexuality. Sexual minority students are simultaneously damaged by official silence and harassing talk. Official silence in curricula gives them no way to adequately address the homophobic words from other students and school professionals. Harassing talk appears to be the source of their problems, but attention to harassment only leaves most official silence in place. In contrast to quick fixes such as speech codes, lack of representation in curricula and lack of advocacy by authority figures are harder to solve by rules that govern individual conduct. So while prohibiting disrespectful speech is the quickest way for school districts to do something, those codes in and of themselves are insufficient. More problematically, policies purportedly intent on protecting sexual minorities from harassment are increasingly being used and interpreted to exclude gay and lesbian issues from public schools. Too often the careful choreography of civil speech is the only action taken to change the school environment. While some speech is stifled, exclusions in curricula, educational and social resources, continue to be clearly heard, felt, and experienced by students of all sexualities.

Because codes of civility and conduct are so closely linked with the practice of propriety, these codes maintain relations of dominance by shifting the focus on structural inequities to matters of social interaction. I am not arguing that structural inequities and social interaction are disconnected but rather that codes of conduct sidestep the material inequalities and install instead a civil place where the difficulties of inequality purportedly do not matter as much as they do in other spaces. Uncivil speech becomes the site of inequalities and thus the place where policy directs its attention. Policies make the individual's speech the focus of concern and thus lodge agency fully within the speaker. As Butler argues, "Such a reduction of the agency of power to the actions of the subject may well seek to compensate for the difficulties and anxieties produced in the course of living a contemporary cultural predicament in which neither the law nor hate speech are uttered exclusively by a singular subject" (1997, p. 80). While it may be difficult to trace the multiple workings of power through a variety of institutions and relations that form bias, it is not so difficult to find the representation of bias within a single speech act. So codes are intent on finding and stopping uncivil speech and also intent on establishing a civil community by removing that offensive speech.

The civility installed by speech codes and other school conduct policies maintain the individual speaker as a source of inequalities and, by suggesting alternative forms of engagement for all participating in the school community, essentially advocate not only fighting speech with speech. Policies intent on forming civil subjects advocate fighting the representation of political inequalities by the practice of social propriety. Civility, then, is a practice that masks differences, not a practice that enables discourse across difference. Further, practices of civility, such as using the correct words to address minority groups and using sensitive language, enable dominant people to protect their own property interest in the source of their dominance. By keeping up the appearance of being cultivated and sensitive, they seem less culpable for inequalities. By gaining a sense of themselves as having currency with issues of diversity, they maintain the veneer of a cosmopolitan person in the know, a kind of tourist of inequality who need never fully engage with the degree to which their own property and investment in saying the right words maintains the inequalities they can converse their way around. In short, speech and conduct codes only keep up the appearance of equality and encourage people to believe that they have, in fact, challenged inequality by using the right words, but not substantially altering their practices. Antidiscrimination policies and speech codes, then, shut down more than offensive speech; these policies prevent education on contentious issues. Further, as if the individual agent fails to behave correctly, the power to adjudicate disturbances falls to the state. As Butler argues, "the state produces hate speech" and thus that speech becomes regulated by the state in ways that reinforce the relations of power between the individual and the state in problematic ways (1997, p. 83). The state will not only not act in the best interests of those harassed, its power will create categories of protection and identity, and conditions for that protection that will be difficult to negotiate.

In at least two states, Massachusetts and Maryland, laws attempting to protect gay and lesbian students from harassment have been crafted specifically to prohibit using those laws as an impetus to bring curricular materials positively representing gays and lesbians into public schools. In other words, both states want harassment to be prevented through a kind of tolerance that dare not speak its name in curricula. In Maryland, the State School Board's lawyers have raised concerns that school anti discrimination policies may bring too much information on homosexuality into public schools because of a "technical glitch" in the text of the policy. When an antidiscrimination bill was approved by the General Assembly in 2001 that banned bias against gays and lesbians, the bill emphasized that public schools are "not required to promote any form of sexuality or include any sexual orientation in the curriculum" (Desmond, 2002, p. 2B). Like the Helms Amendment of the 1980s that prohibited federal funds from supporting AIDS education that promoted homosexuality but was only used to keep funding from gay organizations, the Maryland law uses the language of fairness to suggest that no sexual orientation will find a place in the curriculum. Of course, family life classes continue to advocate heterosexual marriage. School board members are caught between trying to protect gay and lesbian students from harassment, as they must do in order to follow the state antidiscrimination policy, and also trying to avoid opening a loop hole that might allow the introduction of gay and lesbian issues into the curricula. As of the summer of 2002, they are working together with lawyers to ensure that their policy does replicate this "glitch" that might bring gay and lesbian issues into the classroom (Desmond, 2002, p. 2B).

The Massachusetts legislature also simultaneously sought to prevent antilesbian, gay, and bisexual discrimination and limit curricular representations of sexual minorities. When it passed an antidiscrimination policy including protection for sexual orientation to its equal educational opportunity law, the legislature included clauses minimizing the degree to which curricula could represent gay and lesbian issues. The state now calls for schools to start "active efforts" to address and prevent discrimination on the basis of sexual orientation. While original drafts of the law called for schools to "counteract" bias found in curricular materials, the state board revised the law to require that schools "provide balance and context" for bias and stereotypes about sexual orientation (Gehring, 2000, p. 23). In other words, although the schools are required to protect students from anti gay bias, they are also required to provide school time for explanations for that bias. In criticizing the call for making sexual orientation a special form of protection requiring opponents to homosexuality to have voice in the curriculum, one advocate for sexual minorities argued, "We don't hear people say we need balanced views of racism" (LaFontaine quoted in Gehring, 2000, p. 23). Further, changes made to the draft of regulations, now state law, removed a requirement for sexual orientation that is still in place for racial minorities and gender: Curricula should "depict individuals of both sexes and from minority groups in 'a broad variety of positive roles'" (Gehring, 2000, p. 23). While curricula must, for instance, use racially, ethnically, and gender diverse examples and representations, there is no requirement that representation of gays, lesbians, bisexuals, or transgender people be incorporated into curricula. If schools do decide to represent sexual minorities, they are also required to represent those who oppose homosexuality. So, despite the policy's intention to be proactive against bias, Massachusetts actually opens school curricula to representations of bias against sexual minorities in order to appear fair. At the very least, these examples show a high level of ambivalence among policy makers who understand schools are open to liability for discrimination against sexual minority youth. At the worst, even inclusive policies reflect a continuing desire to minimize the protections and representations of sexual minorities. Further, by making discrimination against sexual minorities against the rules, but not part of curricula, schools do not need to engage in substantial discussion of why homophobia is so prevalent, what it means to be a sexual minority, and so on. Official silence can continue to do the work of homophobic harassment by trivializing the experiences of sexual minorities and minimizing representation of sexual minority issues.

Bias as Mere Discourtesy

Even school policies fully committed to protecting and representing a broad range of student diversity have run into problems with the courts. A recent decision indicates that concerns about liability in harassment cases will not easily be solved by installing restrictive antiharassment policies that limit speech. In *Saxe v. State College Area School District,* a broadly conceived school antiharassment policy and speech code that protected sexual minority students, among others, was disallowed by a court that construed the range of things considered by the policy to be harassment as too broad. While the court was concerned that the school district had overstepped its power in circumscribing free speech, the complainant in the case was more specifically concerned with curricular representation of homosexuality. Saxe has been quite candid that his intention was to prevent respect for homosexuality from becoming a school issue. Saxe began his case against the school district when he realized they "were trying to promote homosexuality" and the school used a video that was "a positive look at how teachers deal with homosexuality" (Zernike, 2001, p. A10). As his complaint to the court explains, he and his sons "openly and sincerely identify themselves as Christians. They believe, and their religion teaches, that homosexuality is a sin. Plaintiffs further believe that they have a right to speak out about the sinful nature and harmful effects of homosexuality" (Saxe quoted in United States Court of Appeals for the Third District, *Saxe v. State College,* 2001, p. 2). So any code that attempted to regulate community by excluding speech would necessarily exclude Saxe's sons because their religious commitment requires them to speak out against homosexuality.

The Saxe case is part of a larger trend of conservative challenges to multiculturalism, gay-inclusive nondiscrimination policies, and representations of a variety of minority concerns in school and after-school programs. Character education, for instance, has been embraced by conservatives who argue that the historical/political specificity of multicultural education emphasizes social fractures over commonalities. Rather than educating students about oppression, conservatives want to see all children taught values that have no particular context and respect that has no particular aim. Increasingly conservative groups have begun challenging public school policies that teach tolerance. They claim, "Programs to teach tolerance in public schools are actually being used to promote and encourage homosexuality." In the name of tolerance, "homosexual activists have hijacked our schools. If we don't take a stand, we're going to lose this battle" (McCain, 2002, p. A6).

Regardless of Saxe's particular intentions or the conservative backlash against anti discrimination policies, the court ruled against the conduct code because it lacked a distinction between harassing speech and the sort of uncomfortable speech that was not protected by law. As Judge Samuel A. Alito Jr. argued, "previous courts had ruled that harassment statutes were not violated by epithets that injured someone's feelings, or mere 'discourtesy and rudeness'" (United States Court of Appeals for the Third District, *Saxe v. State College,* 2001, p. 7). In other words, the school district had attempted to limit its liability by preventing speech that made students uncomfortable and in the process had extended the definition of discomfort beyond the legal definition of harassment. While the court supported the school district's concern for liability, it argued that school codes cannot be broader than laws against harassment. Thus the court decided that concerns over liability would have been handled by a narrower conduct policy that did conform to already existing harassment law.

The district argued that it was doing more than attempting to avoid liability and that its policy was attempting to encourage the development of a just and equitable school community. The conduct code was meant to go beyond harassment and liability concerns and into more substantial protections for all students. Judge Alito argued that the code "ignores Tinker's requirement that a school must reasonably believe that speech will cause actual, material disruption before prohibiting it." In addition, because the policy covers speech that has both "the purpose and effect" of "interfering with educational performance or creating a hostile environment," it potentially punishes speech that intends to disrupt, but does not actually disrupt (United States Court of Appeals for the Third District, *Saxe v. State College*, 2001, p. 8). Policy cannot punish an intention, only an effect, according to the court. Further,

> because the Policy's "hostile environment" prong does not, on its face, require any threshold showing of severity or pervasiveness, it could conceivably be applied to cover any speech about some enumerated personal characteristics the content of which offends someone. This could include much "core" political and religious speech: the Policy's "Definitions" section lists as examples of covered harassment "negative" or "derogatory" speech about such contentious issues as "racial customs," "religious tradition," "language," "sexual orientation," and "values." Such speech, when it does not pose a realist threat of substantial disruption, is within a student's First Amendment rights. (U.S. Court of Appeals for the Third District, *Saxe v. State College*, 2001, pp. 11–12).

Even granting that the policy in question is quite broad (though its makers argue it is modeled after state and federal policies), "substantial disruption" means that many people would have to take offense before speech could be regulated by school policy. At the moment, homophobia is pervasive in public schools but not yet thought to be sufficient enough disruption that most faculty and administrators do anything at all about it. For sexual minority youth and those perceived to be sexual minority youth, these disruptions are problematic not because they are widely understood to be disruptive but because they are such perfectly normal situations.

While speech codes are the only answer to homophobia and bias, nonetheless, what students learn from codes is that there are some things worth the protections of codes and other things not worthy. Even giving codes their due as ceremonial markers of importance, though, codes themselves are not enough. Codes also, perhaps against the intention of those who design them, teach that following the code is equivalent to negotiating the difficulties of community and diversity. The code stands for the kind of interactions that might take place under the code and thus can encourage the lazy to go no further than installing a code. In Maryland and Massachusetts, as I described earlier, antidiscrimination policies not only stand in for more substantial education of the school community, but also prohibit more substantial curricular coverage of gay and lesbian issues. Simply providing a policy of protection from discrimination does not, after all, end discrimination. There is a loud silence in curricula that indicates to all students that there are some people in the school who do not deserve to be spoken about and that even some interested in protecting sexual minority youth appear willing to use a community agreement on civil silence as protection.

While educational environments should be challenging and contentious places, it remains striking that opponents to the inclusion of anti gay discrimination clauses in school policies are not interested in making schools easier for sexual minority youth or places where bias is critically examined. The attempted inclusions I have described require as much exclusion as they attempt to prevent. The *Saxe* decision helps provide justification for further exclusions by conceiving of homophobia as trivial rudeness. Calling oppression rudeness and discourtesy misses the historical fact that exclusions are the stuff of courtesy, not rudeness. Civility has historically and contemporarily meant "not saying all that one wishes to say" or not raising difficult issues in a context where there will be disagreement. Under civility's dulling practice, social fractures continued unabated under a watchful process of removing what can be said. Indeed the conservative right's turn away from tolerance and civility in recent years has been in response from the left's attempt to refigure tolerance and civility as inclusion of issues that would previously have been considered inappropriate for polite company. So trying to untangle oppression from public interactions via civility and speech codes uses a tool inappropriate to the task of inclusion and definitely a tool that makes difference, even contentiously debated and intentionally provocative forms of difference, the domesticated stuff of deracinated interaction.

The problem for schools attempting to avoid liability for sexual minority students' (or any students') harassment means that schools must to forge codes that do not upset the school's usual silence on lesbian, gay, bisexual and transgender people. The bind is a difficult one largely because tolerance or civility, if unspecified by class or target, provide no particular coverage. However, as the school district found in *Saxe*, an over specification may mean that school policy extends coverage for students beyond what is reflected in law. The school attempted to argue that this overextension is a good thing because schools are particularly fragile places whose mixture of diversity and youth requires a higher standard of conduct than antiharassment laws. Still, concern with liability or desire to stop harassment through simple codes do not fully educate about and against bias. It is not enough to stop bad words, education is also about explaining and exploring why homophobic bias has so prominent a place in public schools. Covering over the simmering homophobia by making sure students stop using homophobic language in front of teachers would be an improvement, of course, but it not a solution to the problem of near total official silence on sexuality in public schools.

Say the Magic Words

Official silence makes schools hostile places for sexual minority youth and any youth perceived to be a sexual minority. The 2001 Gay Lesbian and Straight Educators Network survey on school climate has found that 99.9% of students surveyed reported hearing homophobic remarks in school (Kosciw & Cullen, 2001, p. 7). Further, homophobic words also damage students of all sexualities, making them cautious about their behavior for fear of being called lesbian or gay. According to the American Association of University Women, being called gay is the only form of harassment that affects boys and girls nearly equally, with 74% of boys and 73% of girls reporting that being called gay or lesbian would make them feel "very upset" (American Association of University Women, 2001, p. 1). What should be clear from these examples is that official silence on lesbian, gay, bisexual, and transgender youth occurs in a climate of constant harassment and speech. Unfortunately, though, the seriousness of that speech or understanding of its nuances is often lost on school authorities.

In a survey I did of school administrators about the school climate for sexual minority students, one principal reported that he had heard anti-gay comments but that they were usually among redneck friends insulting one another, so could hardly be the sort of speech that could be prevented. In addition, he indicated that these words were also not the sort of words anyone would consider insulting because they were clearly directed at friends, even if the intention was to tease those friends. Later, in an interview, another school administrator made a similar comment about the context of "homophobic" slurs at his school. The words "faggot" and "homo" were frequently tossed about among friends, but like the earlier comments on the survey he contended that no one would take them to be serious insults because they were directed only at friends. However, whether the words were directed at friends or not, students know which words to choose to inflict harm. Even if friends use the words to tease one another, other students may understand the content of that teasing differently.

It is not difficult to imagine that a sexual minority student overhearing comments made among friends insulting one another and getting a fairly clear sense that being a "faggot" or "homo" was not something to which one should aspire. Add to that situation the fact that teachers and administrators stop students from using some terms of derision, but allow (and even use themselves) words that insult sexual minorities, and all students learn that some insults are appropriate. When "insults" are appropriate, in fact, they are no longer insults, but rather acceptable ways of describing people one does not like. Banning the use of a word or even broadly suggesting in a code that all students should be tolerated does not guarantee that the experience of the school climate improves, especially if nothing else really changes. If teachers and administrators remain uncomfortable bringing issues affecting sexual minority youth (and any youth who may be interested, which seems likely to be all) into the curricula or if they continue practices that discriminate, restricting speech only masks the degree to which the context has not changed. Suppose that teachers, administrators, and students very earnestly police one another's speech without a full understanding of the complexity and diversity of sexual minority youth. One can imagine a situation in a school with a strict speech code where one young gay man could affectionately call another young gay man a "faggot" and be found to have violated the code. It may be the case, in this imaginary scenario, that the students are punished because of the possibility that other listeners may not have understood the affection with which the term was used. At that point, one rather imagines that the code was doing far too much work and other members of the school community far too little.

In other words, focusing too much on what a nondiscrimination policy or conduct code "does" and not enough on what one might want one's school community to become means that the play of meanings and spaces for different kinds of communication will be diminished. Further, codes with strict and concretized categories of protection may impede the ability of members of the school community to understand variations and innovations that exceed categories they have only tentatively begun to understand. When a gay student at a Chicago school put on high heels for a few minutes, he was told to dress appropriately for his gender or to leave school. While the school has a policy protecting gay students from discrimination, it also has a gender-specific dress code. While the student appears not to identify as transgender, nor does the school have a policy protecting transgender students, it is not fully clear that a policy in and of itself would support this student. Further, the situation raises the question of what sort of policy would best protect this student who clearly understands himself to be more complex than the categories that might protect or expel him. As he explains, "I identify as whatever I put on in the morning" (anonymous student quoted in Barlow, 2002, p. 2). By guaranteeing protection via categories, then, codes allow people to avoid having to fully understand the complexity of their world and consider how categories are constantly complicated by the variety of practice.

Codes also allow people the comfort of falling back on a few conversational techniques to make up for their loss of experience. When asked what they would do if an elementary school child called another child "faggot," my preservice teachers quickly fall back on, "I would tell them that word is inappropriate." They cannot easily say why the word is inappropriate and can, after a little prodding, recall that being told something they were doing was "inappropriate" really did not settle the issue for them when they were kids. However, they are more comfortable dealing with difficult issues if there is a rule to back them up because the rule gets them off the hook for providing an explanation. In short, following a very good understanding of cultural attitudes about homosexuality, students combine their desire to squelch homophobia with a desire to curtail any discussion of queer people. "Inappropriate" is as closely linked to homophobia as it is to homosexuality. Further, "inappropriate" means that the less said about the insulting words, the better. Homophobic incidents become unremarkable in the sense that they will not be remarked upon. Students also say, "the kids don't even know what those words mean," but they also do not want to be the people who provide meaning to the words. They just want the words to be stopped, as if the context for speaking those words is challenged by challenging a speaker without explanation.

Knowing the right rule or the right term replaces fuller discussions of why words cause problems in the first place. A few of my students have, in all seriousness, asked me if it is acceptable to call a Jewish person a Jew because they have only ever heard the word "Jew" as an insult. Likewise, students forced to sit through antihomophobia workshops have often asked if it is ok for them to refer to gays and lesbians as "queers" because they have heard the word used among sexual minorities as a positive term. While I usually say something overly simplistic like, "as long as you don't shout it out of a pick-up truck while tossing a beer bottle, sure, it's ok," the question still sets up the problem of how much context, speaker, and intention go into making words mean something. And even then, the meaning still is not certain. What may set one person's teeth on edge, whoever says it, however it is said, may cause another person no trouble at all. However, students who have little experience with a variety of people from a variety of different groups and background have no way, in their own limited experience, to navigate the complexity and possibility of language. "Experience," of course, is no less complicated than tolerance or meaning, and having the experience of understanding that some things are worthy of being covered by codes and other things are not in themselves instructive experiences, whether one rebels, assents, or continues oneself to grapple with the possibilities.

In these examples of students looking for the right words to say to others, one gets the feeling that the correct words have a magical quality that will heal the social fractures that maintain difference. In discussions with preservice teachers trying to strategize how they would handle a range of bias-related harassment, many students explained that they would be afraid to say the wrong words and thus be mistaken for a racist or a homophobe. They said they would be reluctant to intervene in conflicts between students and even more reluctant to say anything to an overtly biased colleague because their own inexperience with words would indict them as well. The upshot of the discussions has been that until preservice teachers feel comfortable using words associated with diversity, they claim they will not intervene. This dodging of responsibility often travels with exasperated comments like, "I don't know what 'they' want to be called now, it seems like it's always changing and if you call 'them' the wrong thing, 'they'll' get mad." In other words, preservice teachers know what not to say, but because they have likely lived under codes, but not had substantial engagement with diversity or education about diversity, they cannot add to a situation. They can only frustratedly subtract words or phrases that presumably they used to use (or they would not be frustrated) but have now found out are taboo.

Most troubling, like the old "What is a kike? A Jewish gentleman who has left the room," the desire to use the right words only comes up in examples where the group being described is present. The etiquette implied by the necessary presence of the other contains within its restraint the continued presence of suppressed bias. Finding the right words only requires a momentary abatement of the business as usual bias. Part of the frustration of majority students who feel they are being unreasonably asked to curtail their speech or alter their word choice is that they cannot see any real change in not saying all they would like to say. Perhaps because they have lived under school codes and relatively silent curricula, students have learned that changing the words one calls another person counts as sufficient.

Answering Silence with Silence

Sexual minority youth and their allies have used the climate of silence to their own advantage in the most popular antihomophobia demonstration in public schools, the "Day of Silence." Annually, on or about April 9, participants in the "Day of Silence" take a nine-hour vow of silence. They use this time to mark the institutional and personal silences that frame their lives by handing out cards that explain their silence:

> Please understand my reasons for not speaking today. I support lesbian, gay, bisexual, and transgender rights. People who are silent today believe that laws and attitudes should be inclusive of people of all sexual orientations. The Day of Silence is to draw attention to those who have been silenced by hatred, oppression, and prejudice. Think about the voices you are not hearing. (Day of Silence Project, 2001, p. 1)

Information on the Day of Silence suggests that activism is not enough because "actions are too detached from students' daily life. Homophobes can just avoid rallies. Educational events end up preaching to the converted" (Day of Silence Project, 2001, p. 2). However, by being visible about their silence, organizers explain that "everywhere participants go, they are silent in a visible manner to show that they will no longer stand for the silencing of queer people" (Day of Silence Project, 2001, p. 3). While a cynical response to the popularity of this demonstration might be that it is about the least disruptive demonstration one can think of, there is more going on than silence as usual. Intentional silence with the clear purpose of pointing out the normal silencing of sexual minorities seems to raise quite a bit of ire. At my university, the student queer group received numerous claims of harassment from nonally straight people. Apparently being reminded that lesbian, gay, bisexual, and transgender people were specifically deciding not to talk was just too much for a few straight people who had gotten used to not thinking about the fact that queer people were usually silent. One student said she felt "bombarded" by the queer students handing out cards explaining why they were not talking. The effects of silence, then, can be just as troubling as effects of speech. On the one hand, the student was disturbed and thus presumably thinking differently about homophobia. At the same time, though, she had converted the disruption back into a self-centered response. However, that is the danger with using passive aggressive techniques to make a substantive point.

Still, the demonstration gets people thinking and talking about why they had not previously noticed the silence of sexual minorities. In some schools, teachers and nonsilent students have spontaneously engaged in discussions about homophobia. Although one might also be troubled by the fact that the absence of sexual minority voices spurs this conversation on, the Day of Silence action requires that those who normally ignore the situation take more responsibility for their ignorance. Because I am of the generation that preferred yelling in the streets to silence, I worry that the lack of speech allows for a queer-sanctioned "homophobia as usual" and allows too many people to dodge behind the silence as if nothing were happening. Even so, the action does generate response. Media coverage uses the opportunity to provide balanced coverage of conservatives, interviewing protestors, or even seeking out representatives of conservative organizations who had never heard of the protest but, wryly, approve. As one conservative explained to a reporter, "We figured if they're going to be silent, it's a chance for us to speak up even more" (Ovadal quoted in Williams, 2002, p. 1).

Media coverage also takes the opportunity to run its fair share of humorous headlines, like "Shutting Up to Get a Point Across," "Day of Silence Makes Noise," and "Day of Silence Speaks Volumes." In Salt Lake City, where years of court battles ended with the official recognition of the right of Gay Straight Alliances to meet in public schools, coverage of the event mimics homophobic prejudice. "In the past 24 hours, a group of Highland High School students may have heard classmates use such words as 'gay' or 'ghetto' in derogatory ways, make sexist jokes or shun others for their clothing. They didn't say a word to stop it. And that's a good thing." The article goes on to explain that the silence is an action against oppression (May, 2002, p. 1). So one odd effect of the Day of Silence is that non allies are startled to see a silenced minority using passive aggressive techniques to counter its silencing. Whereas the silent treatment may seem initially trivial, the discomfort of students who are not silent grows throughout the day. Silence, in effect, does get their ire up and eventually, like anyone enduring the silent treatment, they have to start asking questions. More than a few participants have explained that their vow does not last long because inevitably someone around them will say something that needs to be answered. The silence of queers then becomes something that nonsilent students have to request an end to.

While I do not think one action is the answer to homophobia, in contrast to codes that limit speech in exchange for limited representation, the Day of Silence highlights institutional, cultural, and personal practices that allow people to remain ignorant of the homophobia structuring their lives. In effect, the intentionality of silence disturbs people who are used to having silence on sexual minorities be the seemingly unintentional norm. If they get to the point where the disruption of homophobia as usual bothers them, they start asking questions of people with whom they may never have spoken or whom they may never have thought might be critical of homophobia. Silence itself is not the whole point of the day, though students do begin to get an idea of the discomforting pervasiveness of silence on sexual minorities. Unlike the tendency of codes to concentrate on individual speech acts as the site of bias, silence shows the pervasiveness of bias, the way silences structure the lives of people, many policies appear on protecting through limitations on speech. The greater point may be that silence has to be addressed and that realization reminds all involved that they are to some degree involved in one another's lives and need to examine uncomfortable and too comfortable silences.

References

American Association of University Women. (2001). *Hostile hallways: Bullying, teasing, and sexual harassment in school.* Accessed at http://www.aauw.org/2000/hostile.html.

Barlow, G. (2002, July 31). Principal gives high heels on boys the boot. *Chicago Free Press.* Accessed at http://www.glsen.org/templates/news/record.html?section=12&record=1386.

Butler, J. (1997). *Excitable speech: A politics of the performative.* New York: Routledge.

Day of silence project. (2001). Accessed at www.glsen.org/templates/student/record.html?section=108&record=636

Desmond, S. (2002, 27 June). School board defers vote on policy to protect gay students. *Baltimore Sun,* 27, p. 2B.

Gehring, J. (2000, 17 May). Mass. stance on anti-gay bias in schools stirring debate. *Education Week,* p. 23.

Kosciw, J. G., & Cullen, M. K. (2001). *The GLSEN 2001 national school climate survey: The school-related experiences of our nation's lesbian, gay, bisexual, and transgender youth.* New York: Gay, Lesbian, and Straight Educators Network.

May, H. (2002, May 30). Highland students use silence to speak out against oppression. *Salt Lake Tribune.* Accessed at http://www.glsen.org/templates/news/record.html?section=12&record=1341.

McCain, R. S. (2002). Tolerance in schools a homosexual ploy, conservatives say. *The Washington Times,* p. A6.

United States Court of Appeals for the Third District. (2001). *David Warren Saxe v. State College Area School District,* No 99–4081.

Williams, S. (2002, April 11). Day of silence disrupted by protests. *Journal Sentinel,* Accessed at: http://www.glsen.org/templates/news/record.html?section=12&record=1296.

Zernike, K. (2001, February 16). Free-speech ruling voids school district's harassment policy. *New York Times,* A10.

PART II

Complicating Speech and Silence

Suzanne deCastell

No Speech Is Free: Affirmative Action and the Politics of Give and Take

Central to the argument of Megan Boler's powerful, provocative, and stimulating essay is its call for an historicized ethics that "recognizes the need to develop ethical principles that take into account that all persons do not have equal protection under the law nor equal access to its resources." In Stanley Fish's words, it is "The sleight-of-hand logic that first abstracts events from history and then assesses them from behind a veil of willed ignorance" (1993) that bolsters anti-affirmative action arguments and legitimizes the perpetuation of institutional inequalities. The pedagogical practices to which historicized ethical principles ought to give rise, Boler argues, are practices of affirmative action applied to classroom speech. Affirmative action pedagogy, she writes, "ensures critical analysis within higher education classrooms of any expression of racism, homophobia, anti-Semitism or sexism," that she further characterizes as "ignorant expressions rooted in privilege." "An affirmative action pedagogy," Boler explains, seeks to ensure that we bear witness to marginalized voices in our classrooms. . . . No utterance that assumes the inferiority of targeted groups is sacred or immune to interrogation" (Boler, this volume).

However, what is meant by *voices* here, and is it the substance of what is spoken, or is it the identity of the speaker that constitutes the basis of differentiated rights to speak? *Voices* is a term that spans these two very different things: A minority student can speak with a racist voice; and the paradigmatic straight white male can voice principles and practices of equity and social justice. And neither has a monopoly on ignorance.

Whether restricting rights to speak is the way to secure freedom to speak is, of course, the trickiest question here, especially if we believe, as the American Civil Liberties Union does, that bigoted speech is only a symptom of a far greater social and cultural problem that is bigotry itself. The discourse of "political correctness" is spoken invariably by those for whom it is merely a troublesome inconvenience that, however, is fairly easily dealt with. Exemplary of this easy solution is the student overheard to say to a peer "I wrote the political correctness section and I guess I'll put it in at the end." We all know we can regulate our speech, but changing our attitudes and actions is another matter altogether. Practices of politeness, whether merely social, or whether indeed enshrined in policy, surely do not amount to the virtues we as educators might wish were their actual motivation. Bernard Williams develops an argument with respect to tolerance that is worth considering in the present context: One possible basis for an attitude of tolerance, "but only one," Williams stresses, is a virtue of tolerance that emphasizes "the moral good involved in putting up with beliefs one finds offensive . . . [but] it is a serious mistake to think that this virtue is the only, or perhaps the most important, attitude on which to ground practices of toleration (Williams, 1996, p. 19). Tolerance as a practice, Williams points out, may most often be grounded in moral indifference, and so, I suggest, might practices of affirmative action in the classroom. So, one line of questioning to pursue here is about whether this essay is proposing an entirely political solution to a largely educational problem, that is not to deny significance to the convergence of the two domains, but nevertheless to insist on significant areas of distinctiveness between education and politics to which educational philosophers should attend.

Of particular historical interest here is how the progressive left has altered in its relation to the issue of freedom of speech: Just a few decades ago, the struggle was for, as de Certeau puts it, the "Capture of Speech," the right to freedom of expression. In more recent years, however, we have seen the progressive left turn increasingly to *restrictions* on speech rights. Why have we found free speech so unruly? How does our conception of violence alter when we shift critical attention from state violence to the violence of citizens toward minority group members, and presume the state to be its neutral arbiter?

Arguing a position in many ways diametrically opposed to the arguments of Boler's paper, Michel de Certeau contends that

> Relations among groups are conflictual by nature. It is thus impossible to subscribe to the idealistic views that assume that conflicts can be resolved by means of a mutual "understanding" or merely by a technical improvement in pedagogical methods. In fact, technical improvement conceals the power that one group exerts over others by defining in its own terms the protocols of the encounter. (de Certeau, 1998, p. 161)

de Certeau calls this strategy an "*ethnicization of political problems*" (p. 162), and calls for an explicitly political clarification and expression that is not constrained by, in his words again, the "obsession with unity," and he urges, in the context of courses on civic morality within a "school for diversity," action and reflection to counteract this "ethnicization" of the political.

The resourcefulness of minority speakers confronted by the apparatuses of power within which they must simultaneously speak against that power, I suggest, is not better served by one particular form of speech over another, and above all it is diminished and not elevated by special rights to speak granted by those same apparatuses.

Writing here on the politics of speech specifically from the standpoint of the revolt of workers and students in France in May and June of 1968, de Certeau stresses the significance of what he terms "the capture of speech." The very idea of a "capture" of speech is significant. Speech was not granted; it was, indeed, captured. Much was risked; struggles ensued—in the streets and universities, to be sure, but also within individuals, in families, between friends, within communities. Speech was not given, it was taken, and this, I think, is important. Because so long as power and participation are granted to its traditional outsiders by those who own the keys to the institution, the risk is that, in de Certeau's words, ". . .the dominant group would be given the dominant role as the essential actor in history" (an actor who becomes, de Certeau adds, "an evil agent if it cannot be a benevolent hero" (1998, p. 162). So seen, even this right to speak is granted under the sign of passivity.

Here again it becomes important to ask: Does this pedagogy accord rights to speak on the basis of what is said or on the basis of who says it, on the basis, that is, of identity? Because of course identities are more often hybrid than pure. More important, identities that are ascribed rather than asserted work, again, to position the subject under the sign of passivity—the teacher, but not I myself, knows who and what I am.

I am troubled, too, by an apparent lapse of historical memory in sentences such as "the uniqueness of classrooms is that, ideally, they provide a public space in that marginalized and silenced voices can respond to ignorant expressions. . . ." Ideally, they do, which is part of the problem with philosophical analysis that forgets its history. How can we forget that the uniqueness of classrooms, *historically*, is that they have effectively accomplished and authorized social relations of hierarchy and subordination, that they have provided a public space for the exercise of power and the legitimizing of racism and oppression in the name of truth, rationality, justice? And, it is in these very same spaces that we will now conduct education as a practice of freedom? How can this happen? By means of what tools can so radical a structural reorganization be accomplished?

When Boler characterizes the to-be prohibited forms of speech as those that "are supported by dominant cultural values institutionalized and validated through social, legal, and political practices" does she forget that education is precisely one such institution? Why place into the mouths of students institutionally supported racism, sexism, homophobia, and so on, as if these students were their originary speakers, rather than words ventriloquized by subordinated subjects of the school's, and later the university's epistemological and ethical "canon," its "official knowledge" about its proper subjects, and its proper subject matters. If our students were the *source* of such ignorance and hostility, rather than merely the enunciators of what schools and universities have taught them, we might hope to deploy schools and universities as gatekeepers in practices of their eradication. However, if students are merely the mouthpieces for the official discourse that protects and preserves a political condition of radical social inequality, do we not, as Judith Butler (1997) warns, unwittingly suspend critical insight into state power and state violence when we displace power and violence onto individual citizens of whose rights to speak the state is thereby constituted as neutral arbiter?

If we are presupposing in such an argument that teachers are willing and able to transform pedagogy by means of critical dialogue, why do we do so? What theory of change is at work here?

The Talking Cure

It is at this point that many educational theorists turn to the pre-eminent tool set of subject formation, the practice of speech, and to the particular form of speech privileged by educators since Socrates (and no less spurious today than in his time), that distinctive set of deceptions and deformations we like to call "dialogues." Why has such passionate effort been devoted to defending the sanctity of the dialogue as the educative method of choice? I suggest that dialogue does not in fact have the effect it is presumed to have, and at the level of its theoretical conceptualization, we have to ask why so many have made impassioned arguments for it. Recall here Foucault's (1978, 1988) extensive critical interrogations of the obligation to speak, the institutionalizing of the practice of confession, and, of particular importance for educators, its normalizing, in his words, "disciplinary" function.

Indeed Boler's first paragraph announces this: ". . . our social and political culture predetermines certain voices and articulations as unrecognizable, illegitimate, unspeakable." It is ironic indeed, then, that the argument following this acknowledgment of historically prestructured inequalities of speaking is an argument for the special protection of rights to speak. What kind of right is this right to deliver unrecognizable utterances always already illegitimately spoken by unspeakable subjects—and how can it be enforced and defended?

More important for my purposes is the presupposition too often made with respect to the talking cure—the insistence that hearing silenced voices, by that of course we mean people talking—fixes everything. I am not even sure whether talking fixes anything—but certainly talking does not "fix" social injustice even within the microcosm of the classroom, let alone fixes what is at root a political-administrative and not an ethical or an educational problem. In fact, as Butler (1997) has argued, prohibiting hostile speech cannot be done except by re-citing it, and in that re-citation, the possibility of repeating its harms is ever present.

One right that educators ought not to defend, however, is the right to be ignorant and the right to speak ignorantly. And this is not specific to any particular community or type of student or type of speech. If educators refused that right of ignorance to their students, wouldn't pretty much all the kinds of speech that affirmative action pedagogy seeks to prohibit by resorting to speech codes be dealt with? What kinds of undesirable speaking would be left over?

Teaching often will involve, indeed necessarily does involve, the temporary, tactical, and selective suppression and privileging of what students might wish to say. But in the end, educating is the job of the educator, and what gets said in the classroom may be more important than whether or not it is the students themselves who say it.

While the First Amendment prohibits the making of *laws* restricting freedom of speech, and that prohibition does make any attempt to violate freedom of speech a risky business, there is no constitutional requirement for educators to afford full rights to speak to all students at all times, and indeed they have never done so. What we see here is not the courageous educator seeking equity and social justice even at the risk of breaking the law, but, sadly and pathetically enough, the too frequent timidity of educators who clutch at the First Amendment as a justification for *not* doing what they ought to do, and saying what they ought to say, even though their freedom of speech is protected.

Instead of criticizing ethically impoverished practice, shall we say to teachers "You will be entitled to silence students who oppose you, if you feel intimidated about affirming equity and inclusion, we will create a team of allies who will speak on your behalf. If you feel too exposed, you need not risk disclosure of your own otherness, we will find a majority speaker whose voice secures for you protective coloration . . . you can be a coward, weak, closeted, and we will make it possible for you to be an activist for social justice." Meanwhile, what work are we doing to afford protection to those far less powerful Others whom we would encourage to speak their difference, by a temporary and artificially enclosed silencing of otherwise dominant peers?

The truth is, whatever arguments we can marshal, teachers, and especially women and minority teachers, are rarely *able* in reality to silence speech both hostile *and* ignorant, when spoken by dominant "voices." Given our inability to create adequately protected discursive environments, why is so much attention paid to protecting the educator from the dangers of practicing equity and inclusion, and why is so little attention paid to making practices of equity and inclusion less dangerous for students of a different "voice"? For it is not at all clear to me that protecting the first secures the last.

References

Boler, M. (This volume). All speech is not free: the ethics of "affirmative action pedagogy."

Butler, J. (1997). *Excitable speech: A politics of the performative.* London: Routledge.

De Certeau, M. (1998). *The capture of speech.* Minneapolis: University of Minnesota Press.

Fish, S. (1993). Reverse racism, or how the pot got to call the kettle black. *www.Theatlantic.com/ politics/race/fish.htm*

Foucault, M. (1978). *The history of sexuality* (Vols. 1–3) (R. Hurley, Trans.). New York: Random.

Foucault, M. (1988). Technologies of the self. In L. Martin, H. Gutman, & P. Hutton (Eds.), *Technologies of the self: A seminar with Michel Foucault* (pp.16–49) Amherst: University of Massachusetts Press.

Williams, B. (1996). Toleration: An impossible virtue? In D. Heyd (Ed.), *Toleration: An elusive virtue.* Princeton: Princeton University Press.

Alison Jones

Talking Cure: The Desire for Dialogue

In her notes to contributors, Megan Boler posed to the writers of this book what she called its "central questions":

> What challenges of voice/speaking/dialogue arise in your teaching practice? Is democratic dialogue possible in our classrooms? Is it a worthy ideal? How do existing social inequalities make dialogue problematic? Should certain forms of speech and/or certain historically constructed identities or voices be "privileged" as a form of historical redress?

What is this desire for dialogue? Why should we want to talk to each other? The commonsense answer is that it has to be a good thing to be able to communicate across difference. In its ideal form, dialogue between diverse groups dispels ignorance about others, increases understanding, and thus potentially decreases oppression, separation, violence, and fear.

The calls for communication between ethnic groups seem to be more urgent since the events of September 11, 2001. If it was already a good idea before the al-Qaeda attacks on New York and Washington to establish genuine cross-cultural dialogue, its importance certainly intensified afterwards. Conversation between adversaries, or just between those of different racial and religious backgrounds, is seen increasingly as a social good, at least by those seeking a peaceful means of resolving difference or conflict. Dialogue, it is assumed, provides the opportunity for the development of tolerance, understanding, and ultimately unity; it can decrease instances of ignorance and racism and other prejudices that are the basis of social division. Not only will dialogue between groups decrease actual threat, but also—insofar as it leads to the dominant group knowing more about the other—it potentially reduces imagined threat by improving social cohesion.

While the paragraphs above are littered with controversial claims and assumptions, I do not examine these here. I am interested not in the justification, potential benefits or processes of dialogue, but in the apparently innocent and well-intentioned desires for dialogue in educational settings. If some practical justification for my interest is required, I would suggest that identification of the common fantasies swelling these desires might ease the disappointments that inevitably arise when dialogue does not quite work.

Classrooms, Voice and Dialogue

Democratic classrooms have long been seen as a key training ground for the urgent social good called cross-cultural dialogue. What such an important practice might look like in action regularly remains unexplained, but dialogue in educational settings is usually understood in terms of members of different groups (typically at odds in terms of beliefs or social positioning, or from different cultural communities) communicating directly with one another through speech. School environments are often more ethnically diverse than other sites, and young people from different groups are bought together into close contact not found elsewhere. Therefore, classrooms are seen to offer an excellent opportunity for the guided development of good cross-cultural communication skills, as well as the chance to learn about, and from, one another.

For progressive educators, particularly at the university level, such communication is not merely an exercise in "learning more about our world." Talking together is a truly progressive educational exercise that offers to promote identification with others and to create a less divided and ultimately more just society. While there are many divergent views among tertiary-level educators and academics about what counts as dialogue, how it might occur and what might be its possibilities, it is largely seen as a practice central to social justice and democracy.

The key idea in contemporary praise of dialogue in education is voice—or speech—which is set in opposition to silence. We are exhorted to "hear the voices" of those who have previously been silent. In a democratic classroom, those who do not usually speak are provided with opportunities to have their voices heard. Megan Boler, for instance, asks that we

> bear witness to marginalized voices in our classrooms . . . The uniqueness of classrooms is that, ideally, they provide a public space in which marginalized and silenced voices can respond. . . . The classroom is one of the few public spaces in which one can respond and be heard. (Boler, this volume)

Thus democratic dialogue is far more than an opportunity for the exchange of ideas, or gathering interesting information about other people's lives. It is an explicitly political event because it attempts to shift the usual flow of power in order to un-marginalize the marginalized. Voices that are usually marginalized—which is to say silenced—are to be centered and therefore empowered.

Of course, how such centering or demarginalization might occur is the difficult question. Undeterred, progressive educators in the last ten or fifteen years have called for diverse groups of students to engage in "affirming and celebrating the interplay of different voices and experiences," so that worthwhile education and emancipatory politics can be "created out of empathy for others by means of a passionate connection through difference" (McLaren, 1995, pp. 40, 160). In democratic classrooms, transparency, communication, and accessibility are the basic educational skills. Uncomfortable silences, negative comments, prejudice, and lack of interest in the other—the taints of colonization and subordination, and lack of mutual understanding—are to be challenged (Aronowitz & Giroux, 1991). This challenge is both to the prejudices and stereotypes spoken by those who usually speak, and to the silence of the marginalized. Progressive educators desire to "hear the voices" of the oppressed/other (Aronowitz & Giroux, 1991, p. 129), as they "invite [these] students themselves to become the mediators of their own narratives" (McLaren, 1995, p. 115) and actors in their own liberation.

The result, as progressive educators put it in the early 1990s, is that both usually dominant and usually silent groups "cross over into realms of meaning . . . that are increasingly being renegotiated and rewritten . . ." (Aronowitz & Giroux, 1991, p. 119). What we might "become together" in such renegotiation, suggests McLaren (1995, p. 109), takes precedence over "who we are." Whether we are women or men, gay or straight, black or white, Muslim or Christian, the shared talk of multiple voices is crucial to progressive pedagogy. With a touching faith in the "talking cure" of dialogue and self-disclosing narrative, emancipatory educators argue that, via a multiplicity of voices/narratives, teachers and students can speak and work across differences towards an egalitarian, multicultural, and democratic social order in the classroom—and elsewhere.

Some progressive educators, including contributors to this volume, take a somewhat more complex view. They focus on the fact that wider social inequalities impact significantly upon the possibilities of shared talk in the classroom. They foreground inequality not as something to be reduced by dialogue, but as a barrier to genuinely productive conversation. They are cautious about utopian fantasies of empathy and unity, and argue for the development of a "dialogic ethics in which classroom conversation can be opened, tested, and redefined among unequally located speakers" who can then work toward coalitions or even separate struggles (Roman, 1993, p. 84). For Boler, as her "central questions" above suggest, such a dialogic ethics might consider the difficult issues of historical redress and the privileging of some traditionally silenced voices over others, rather than encouraging an equal flow of communication both ways.

Even so, what might it mean to "privilege" traditionally marginalized voices? The most obvious reading of this suggestion is that teachers might encourage and enable usually silenced groups to speak out by especially inviting their engagement. In a mixed classroom, this might mean asking the whole group to focus on the views and experiences of one section. It might entail inviting speakers from a marginalized group and requiring engagement from all students, or encouraging the development of caucus groups that would allow the usually marginalized to express themselves from a position of collective solidarity.

A more unpalatable reading of the request to privilege some voices is that in order to foreground some viewpoints, others (hate-filled, or prejudiced, or dominant) must be discouraged, criticized, or silenced. This sort of position, which appears undemocratic because in elevating some voices it demotes or silences others, is avoided by many university teachers. To privilege some voices and not others is considered biased—even "racist" because (white) participants might be silenced on the grounds of ethnicity—not to mention the old liberal view that silencing *any* voice puts freedom of speech under threat.

However one confronts the problems of dialogue and inequality, it is the case that any silence or silencing generates anxiety—both in a dialogic classroom, and in a democratic society which relies on and prizes public, speaking participation.

Disturbing Silence

To a progressive educator, the silence of the other is most disturbing. It seems to signal not only a lack of dialogue but oppression and marginalization. Of course, from the point of view of the silent other, the decision not to speak may be rather less troubling and rather more eloquent than it appears; it may be a pragmatic rejoinder to a set of conditions beyond their control. Silence may be a rational response to their (dominant) peers' lack of ability to hear and understand. Many nonwhite students' views and experiences may not be expressible in the language of the classroom (in which dialogue is conducted), and hence they may choose to remain silent rather than attempt the unspeakable. As the straight-talking Hispana Maria Lugones put it: "We and you do not talk the same language. When we talk to you, we use your language: the language of your experience and of your theories. We try to use it to communicate our world of experience. . . . We cannot talk to you in our language because you do not understand it" (Lugones & Spelman, 1983, p. 575).

Lugones and Spelman's remarks seem to suggest that if "you" cannot understand, in order for dialogue to occur, "you" must be taught, and "we" must teach you. From the perspective of the marginalized, dialogue is beginning to sound very much like difficult teaching. Indeed, from the others' point of view, many of the dominant group are "slow learners" and often very hard to educate—particularly about cultural difference and the effects of power. Given that nonwhite or other minority students seldom have the duty, desire, or ability to take on the task of teaching slow or recalcitrant white classmates, many of them sensibly avoid its demands and remain silent.

Research focused on my Education Studies classes illustrates the notion of nonwhite students' refusal to teach their white peers, and their resistance in the face of the white students' desire to be taught by them (Jones, 1999, 2001). While the silence of nonwhite students in my classes may not have been a conscious strategy of resistance/refusal, it could not be understood merely as a direct product of "being unable to speak," "being silenced," or "not having the opportunity to respond." Many Maori and Pacific students in my university classes lacked the desire to satisfy the curiosity of their white peers who, in the spirit of dialogue, wanted to debate or question their views, or to "know what it is like [being Maori]," or who simply did not understand what the nonwhite students had to say. Many did not want to have to explain when white classmates asked, whether out of genuine curiosity or malevolence: "Why should we learn about Maori things? They are only one small group," or "Maori are always talking about the past. We should all get going towards the future." Most of the Maori and Pacific students refused to provide the pedagogical work required to bring their white peers to a point of basic understanding, acceptance, and empathy so that dialogue could even begin to be a possibility.

In an attempt to experiment with successful education strategies for all students, my Maori teaching colleagues and I separated the students along ethnic lines for some classes. For the nonwhite students, this strategy represented a joyful opportunity; in their own group where others "spoke the same language," their silence was broken and they "felt more confident" and "felt validated." One said the experience "broadened my horizons to question, argue, and debate" (Jones, 1999, p. 303). As their Maori teachers put it: "We were revelling in our space. . . . I don't think the revelry was because we had got a Maori space. The revelry was because the Maori women were controlling the information; they could engage it and suddenly they were being successful" (Jenkins & Pihama, 2001, p. 302). In a separate group, the Maori and Pacific students' pedagogical work was shared work. No longer were they required to be the teachers or providers; they could advance their educational interests in developing their own shared knowledge and internal arguments. Thus, the separation from their white peers was experienced as empowering and positive.

This separation was not welcomed by the white students. The profound silence of the other, created by their absence, was met with anger. Suddenly, the potential providers of knowledge of the other were gone. Many of the white students made such remarks as: "It does not seem right. Could we not learn from each other? Wouldn't it be valuable to share our differences in experience? . . . It is different reading about it in books, or having it taught by teachers. It is better to hear it straight from the women who are having the experience." "Nothing can be changed unless 'we' know and are aware of what needs to be changed. Behind closed doors doesn't help the process of change" (Jones, 1999, p. 302). Curiously perhaps, white students' anger at the loss of this "sharing" was not evident when all the students were together, even though the Maori and Pacific students tended not to share their differences in experiences with their white peers in the mixed class-room. The nonwhite students' (even silent) presence in the classroom was more than acceptable, it was desired; their organized absence was not.

The white students' anger at the disturbing silence/absence of their nonwhite peers is particularly interesting because it is a symbolic indication of what might be at stake, at least for dominant groups, in calls for classroom dialogue. Dialogue is based, however cautiously it might be considered, in a dominant group fantasy or romance about access to and unity with the other. This is the fantasy of a democracy based in consensus reached from rational debates across different views and groups. It is a truly magnificent, if flawed, romantic ideal. Inevitably, anxiety and anger are readily expressed when such a romance appears thwarted or threatened in any way. The loss of the ideal of democratic dialogue and its promise of social cohesion is a serious one; it suggests loss of the basic fantasies on which western democracies are built. Therefore, those with sincere and benevolent desires for a unified and egalitarian classroom and society are likely to identify as a threat any apparently contrary practice such as the withdrawal or active silence of some groups.

The experience of this threat is not uncommon in education, particularly among white people in multicultural settings. Virginia Chalmers (1997) tells a story that illustrates the anxiety and threat felt by some white parents in New York City when she organized a lively evening for parents of color at her school. People of color did not normally come to school meetings, and the separate meeting was an attempt—successful as it turned out—to encourage their participation. The angry reaction of the white parents who were not invited to the meeting was marked by words such as "exclusion" and "loss." Like most of my white students, the white parents in the New York school believed that racial equality and communication could not occur with any separation of ethnic groups. However, for the parents of color, the separation from white people was a necessary strategy to discuss and plan change that would lead, they believed, to improved possibilities for high-quality education for their children—and thus, ultimately, increased equality.

In education, the threat to dialogue has particular emotional force because it is a threat to the dominant group at the very point of their/our power in education—

to their ability to know. A sense of exclusion and outrage marks the refusal of the already privileged to accept that some knowledge and relationships might not be available to them/us. The Enlightenment project of mapping the world, rendering it visible and understood, does more than shape our education system: It is also at the root of the threat we feel when nonwhite peers separate from us, or show little interest in teaching us. Our education system is based in the western desire for coherence, authorization, and control. This desire fuels the calls for democratic dialogue, or hearing the voices of the marginalized. These are in effect calls for access to the other, and to the knowledge and experiences of the other.

Disturbing Absence, Disturbing Presence

In a classroom where nonwhite peers are absent, the possibility of hearing the voices, of access to the marginalized other, is denied to white students. I have suggested that in liberal and progressive educational discourse, the dominant cultural assumption is that access to the other through understanding is integral to a modern, progressive, multiethnic education system, and society. Therefore, the removal of the possibility of gaining knowledge of the other from the other (assured through their presence, and therefore their potential engagement) means that the white students and parents accurately sense a powerful loss.

One might expect, then, that the presence of nonwhite teachers in front of white classes might be helpful to those who are threatened by the loss of their nonwhite peers. In fact, though, for my white students, the Maori and Pacific teachers generated discomfort rather than salvation. Many white students became irritated at the pedagogies of their Maori and other nonwhite teachers, which did not connect with the white students' knowledge and views. In contrast to the Maori students, who often became silent in the face of the white teachers' pedagogy and the questioning and debate of their white peers, the white education students taught by assertive Maori teachers became restless, asked sulky questions, or stayed away, complaining that they had been marginalized. In other words, the privileging of Maori voices of authority produced intense anxiety for many of the white students. When white students had to listen to unfamiliar (Maori) words, or consider their own relationship to Maori things, they felt "marginalized," "tired," "stupid," "uncomfortable," and discouraged (Jones, 2001, pp. 281–282). Their sense of dislocation was sharp as they were suddenly displaced from the unproblematic center of knowing and cut off from access to what counts as knowledge in the university. The shift in boundaries of legitimate knowledge, marked by the Maori teachers' words, was met with confused resistance and dismay. The point is: If the silence of, or separation from, the other is disturbing, access to the other may be even more so.

Providing the white students with nonwhite teachers did not meet the students' desires for access to their peers through dialogue. The fantasy of talking together and the romance of access required the embodied presence of peers, who were available in ways the teacher was not. Did the white students resist the nonwhite teacher because she had the authority to demand the white students' engagement with something they instinctively felt was inaccessible to them? Perhaps the nonwhite peers epitomized the accessible other, in ways that the teacher cannot. If that was the case, it was only the peers' presence that could fulfill the dominant students' fantasy of access to, and understanding of, the other.

I have suggested elsewhere (Jones, 1999) that the desire for the embodied other in the shape of peers may also be a desire for redemption, or forgiveness, on behalf of the white students. The direct (or even silent) attention of nonwhite peers is somehow experienced by the white students as an act of grace ("I care about what you think. I do not really hate you, despite your dominant position") or of forgiveness ("Do not feel badly about my marginalized situation; I hear your anxieties, and your sincere attempts to understand, and I forgive you"). Inchoate desires for redemption and reassurance in an unequal world fuel the desire of the powerful for dialogue.

Dialogue as Colonization

It is clear, then, that while incitement to dialogue might seem, on the surface, to be innocent and neutral, the call for dialogue and shared talk makes very different demands on the two groups involved. My arguments suggest that, paradoxically, progressive teachers' calls for dialogue may to be in danger of reproducing the very power relations they seek to critique. I have suggested that dialogue requires particular pedagogical work from the subordinate group. The other, via voice, must work hard to donate (provide access to) her experience and views to the dominant other.

"Work" is also required of the dominant group—but it is of a particular kind, the kind of work dominant groups can and must do as they unconsciously maintain their position. This is the work of hearing. Calls for democratic dialogue are calls for (and often by) the dominant group to listen, or to hear the voices of the marginalized. After all, listening is hardly required the other way around; members of marginalized/colonized groups do not need to encounter the voice of the powerful—they are immersed in it and hear it daily. Maria Lugones again: ". . . we have had to be in your world and learn its ways. We have to participate in it, make a living in it, live in it, be mistreated in it . . . in learning to do these things . . . we have had to learn your culture and thus your language and self-conceptions" (1997, p. 576; also see Cook, 1997; Essed, 1990). So, even though dialogue-discourse is about hearing each other, it is really about the dominant group hearing the other.

In other words, what is ultimately most significant to dialogue is not the talking by the marginalized, but the hearing by the dominant group. The "actor," or the one who ultimately determines the success or failure of the dialogic encounter, is the dominant group—again. Dialogue and recognition of difference turn out to be access for dominant groups to the thoughts, cultures, lives of others. While marginalized groups may be invited—with the help of the teacher—to make their own social conditions visible to themselves, the crucial aspect of the dialogic process is making themselves visible to the powerful.

If we take seriously Barthes's arguments about the power of the reader to make the text, and his point that understanding "lies not in [a text's] origin but in its destination" (Barthes, 1994, p. 148), then it is not so much the other's voice but its "heard voice," its audience in the classroom, that becomes the key player in meaning. When dominant group members are unable to understand the speaker, because they do not have the "ears to hear" (Babich, 1994, p. 27), then the other's ability (let alone desire) to speak in the classroom must be reduced dramatically—as the Maori and Pacific students in my classes seemed to indicate. In short, when the dominant group cannot hear the marginalized voices, dialogue cannot occur.

What really underlies calls to dialogue is not the dominant group's longing for inclusion of others. Rather, the dominant group seeks its *own* inclusion by being rescued from its inability to hear the voices of the marginalized. It construes silence as the absence of the other's speech, but the silence is in the ears of the powerful— who (mis)recognize it as the silence of the excluded other. Progressive teachers seek to name and repair this exclusion. Even so, paradoxically, the dialogic solution lies in repairing the exclusion of the dominant group, positioning them again in the driver's seat.

Progressive educators would rightly be outraged at any suggestion that the benevolent desire for dialogue might entail unconscious colonizing assumptions. They would emphasize that they seek merely to respect and uphold difference, through having it spoken, shared, and critiqued, where once it was suppressed. While this might seem reasonable on the surface, Homi Bhabha suggests such innocent motives may be more problematic than they seem. Using Derrida's phrase, he talks of the colonizer's demand for narrative, "the narcissistic, colonialist demand it should be addressed directly, that the Other should authorise the self, recognise its priority, fulfil its outlines . . ." (Bhabha, 1994, p. 98). The address of the other involves answering the colonizer's benign, maybe even apologetic, request: "Tell us exactly what happened"; "What is it like for you?" This demand, according to Bhabha, is not an opportunity for subordinate groups to express themselves, enter the conversation, and become empowered, but is a significant "strategy of surveillance and exploitation" and reensures the authority of the colonizer (Bhabha, 1994, pp. 98–99).

Conclusion

Why, then, must the marginalized speak (engage in dialogue)? For whose benefit do they speak? They speak for our benefit in that they meet our desires to understand, and their speech is granted by our hearing. In the talking cure, it is clear that power remains concentrated at the usual places—that is, with the powerful, as they/we attempt to grant subjugated knowledge a voice. The members of the dominant group remain the dominant actors in the dialogic relationship.

In response to my critique of the desire for dialogue, some would agree that dialogue might be for the powerful, in order to inform them—but that there is also an important sense in which it is not only for them, ultimately. When dominant groups gain a better understanding of marginalized groups through dialogic teaching by them, the outcome might be in the interests of the marginalized. To the extent that dialogue results in the reduction of prejudice and ignorance in members of powerful groups, positive social change will ultimately result. When this result occurs, it raises the troubling possibility that dialogue may be understood as a sort of colonization where the powerful require the subordinate to open their territory for exploration (so the powerful can hear the marginalized voices). Armed with this new knowledge, the white knowers will, we are meant to believe, run a more just world. Many indigenous and colonized peoples would attest to the failure of this strategy.

In this view, dialogue can be seen as enervating rather than empowering for nondominant groups. A safer, more productive bet for them would be to shore up their own internal communication and knowledge systems, and from this base struggle for improved social conditions. Such a suggestion tends to be a rather negative response to Megan Boler's questions about the possibility of democratic dialogue in classrooms, and to imply that "challenges to dialogue" are insurmountable. Despite my critical voice, I am reasonably optimistic. With more critical understanding of the complexities and contradictions inherent in apparently benign and progressive desires for dialogue in education, we might reduce our romantic expectations of dialogue, and set about working alongside and with each other in different ways. Dialogue, if it occurs, will most likely be a serendipitous by-product of that more oblique engagement.

One of the characters in the Inuit (Canadian Eskimo) film *Atanarjuat: The Fast Runner* says that he cannot sing his song to those who do not understand it. It has no meaning to them, so why would he sing it? To sing it under such circumstances may even be harmful to the singer, by being misunderstood. This is the deep contradiction at the heart of our desires for dialogue—we cannot hear others if we do not understand them; we cannot understand them unless we can hear others. It is undeniably the case that fantasies and acts of shared communication are preferable to fantasies and acts of ignorance and separation. However, desires for shared communication must be mediated more by cautious critique and limited expectations than by urgent and ultimately self-defeating optimism.

References

Aronowitz, S., & Giroux, H. (1991). *Postmodern education: Politics, culture and social criticism.* Minneapolis: University of Minnesota Press.

Babich, B. (1994). *Nietzsche's philosophy of science: Reflecting science on the ground of art and life.* New York: State University of New York Press.

Barthes, R. (1994). *Image—Music—Text.* New York: Hill and Wang.

Bhabha, H. (1994). *The location of culture.* New York: Routledge.

Boler, M. (This volume). All speech is not free: The ethics of "affirmative action pedagogy."

Chalmers, V. (1997). White out: Multicultural performances in a progressive school. In M. Fine, L. Weis, L.C. Powell, & L. Mun Wong (Eds.), *Off white: Readings on race, power and society* (pp. 66–78). New York: Routledge.

Cook, D. (1997). The art of survival in academia: Black women faculty finding where they belong. In M. Fine, L. Weis, L.C. Powell & L. Mun Wong (Eds.), *Off white: Readings on race, power and society* (pp. 100–109). New York: Routledge.

Essed, P. (1990) *Everyday racism: Reports from women of two cultures.* Alameda, CA: Hunter House.

Jenkins, K., & Pihama, L. (2001). Matauranga Wahine: Teaching Maori women's knowledge alongside feminism. *Feminism and Psychology, 11*(3), 293–303.

Jones, A. (1999). The limits of cross-cultural dialogue: Pedagogy, desire and absolution in the classroom. *Educational Theory, 49*(3), 299–315.

Jones, A. (2001). Cross-cultural pedagogy and the passion for ignorance. *Feminism and Psychology, 11*(3), 279–292.

Lugones, M. C., & Spelman, E.V. (1983). Have we got a theory for you! Feminist theory, cultural imperialism and the demand for "the woman's voice." *Women's Studies International Forum, 6*(6), 573–581.

McLaren, P. (1995). *Critical pedagogy and predatory culture.* London: Routledge.

Roman, L. (1993). White is a color! White defensiveness, postmodernism, and antiracist pedagogy. In C. McCarthy and W. Crichlow (Eds.), *Race, identity, and representation in education* (pp. 71–88). New York: Routledge.

Huey Li Li

Rethinking Silencing Silences

Silence is a complex and complicated cultural phenomenon. While it is common to view silence as the opposite of speech, silence also complements speech. After all, silence and speech form a continuum of human communication. Furthermore, silence can be intentional or unintentional. Intentional silence may be a deliberate cultural practice that aims at facilitating introspection and self-discipline (Greene, 1940; Dauenhauer, 1980). At the same time, the practice of presumably unintentional silence may originate from long-term acculturation and embodies semiotic experiences (Enninger, 1987). Both intentional and unintentional silences have multiple meanings that are open to varied interpretations. In effect, silence is both the signifier and the signified (Kurzon, 1998). Thus, any effort to formulate the final definition of silence can be easily entrapped in an infinite regress of definitions. Instead of searching for a final definition of silence, a critical inquiry into silence should focus on how silence works in different communicative contexts (Jaworski, 1993).

In educational settings, silence plays an important yet ambiguous role in the formation of school culture. On the one hand, it is still a widely accepted belief that silencing is an indispensable disciplinary act that aims at establishing an ordered milieu for effective teaching and learning. Silence as an educational state during a designated period of time thus reveals and sustains hierarchical power relationships. In view of the disciplinary nature of silence, Paulo Freire (1970) argues that "human existence cannot be silent, nor can it be nourished by false words, but only by true words, with which men [*sic*] transform the world" (p. 76). In line with Freire's effort to reconstruct the "culture of silence," many concerned educators have made concerted efforts to unpack and disclose "the multiple forms of public silencing" (Weis & Fine, 1993) that have contributed to sustaining oppressive cultural institutions and practices. To a large extent, these educators recognize silence as both a consequence of and a form of resistance to oppression. Beyond elucidating the structuring of silence, concerned educators are also committed to reclaiming the silenced voices (e.g., Houston & Kramarae, 1991; Zimmerman & Rojas, 1998; Lazreg, 1994). The underlying belief is that the silenced people have the right to speak out and to be heard.

On the other hand, the use of silence in educational settings may simply allow time for reflection on teaching and learning, which further facilitates more meaningful interactions between teachers and students. For instance, wait-time—a moment of silence—can make positive contributions to both teaching and learning (Rowe, 1974). Likewise, a lack of silence often characterizes unsuccessful psychotherapy while silence is an indicator of successful sessions (Cook, 1964). In addition, multicultural education movements have raised many educators' awareness of cross-cultural differences in terms of the use of silence in educational settings. To illustrate, Navajo children are more inclined to learn by silently observing the surrounding world, whereas Euro-American cultures tend to recognize and accept speech as a legitimate and desired form of educational interaction. As educational institutions in the west tend to solemnize the right of speech, it is not surprising that western education systems stress the need to cultivate and test all students' language skills. Consequently, it is easy for teachers to underrate Navajo children's cognitive abilities, owing to their lower verbal test scores (John, 1972; Dumont, 1972).

Because educational discourses on silence as a disciplinary act appear to erroneously render silence as a monolithic psycholinguistic phenomenon, it is not clear whether silencing as a disciplinary act is so powerful that silence is the inevitable consequence of oppression. In other words, the polarizing of the silencers and the silenced seems to oversimplify the power structure within and beyond educational institutions. Moreover, the pedagogical use of silence such as wait-time focuses primarily on the instrumental value of silence as if silence has no intrinsic pedagogical merits. Above all, while many educators have raised their awareness of varied uses of silences in different cultural contexts, educators have yet to undertake a more in-depth inquiry into aims and methods of incorporating multicultural perspectives of silence into educational processes.

In this essay, I first offer a critique of the primacy of speech in modern schooling and call for a recognition of the pedagogical merits of silence in facilitating reflective teaching and learning. Second, I argue that, in forging co-intentional pedagogy as endorsed by Paulo Freire (1970), educators must not deliberately silence silence because silencing silence as an intentional pedagogical act could ratify speech as the privileged form of human communication. Instead, it is essential for educators to question the polarization of silence and speech and to challenge the primacy of speech in current discourse on multicultural education. Beyond reclaiming silenced voices, educators also need to inquire into silence as a source of pedagogical knowledge.

Rethinking Pedagogical Merits of Silence

Speech and silence actually form a continuum of human communication. To a certain degree, the complementary relationship of speech and silence indicates that silence and speech are functionally equivalent. However, such a pragmatic viewpoint concerning the interdependence and inseparability between speech and silence do not therefore suggest that silence and speech have equal values in all cultures. In fact, speech has been the preferred means of communication in most modern societies where technological advancement lures us to eschew silences and to further justify intolerance of silences. The following observation of American culture may be applicable in other industrialized and urbanized societies as well:

> America is a nation of gap fillers and space pluggers. We are individuals who usually do not listen to other people. We talk all the time, even when others are talking. People are deluged by radio and television. We awaken and we go to sleep caught up in gossip, news of violence, and people acting funny interrupted by high-pitched bursts of loud laughter. Our social lives are a mélange of noise. We settle for lighthearted, flickering relationships and recreational sins, and revel in offensive talk on the electronic media carnival. (Wilmer, 2000, p. 19)

As mass media and computer-mediated communication systems constantly erode or even deplete silences at a macro level, it is nearly impossible for individuals to learn to appreciate rare moments of silence. In high paced societies, it is not surprising that very few people are committed to interpreting silence, which demands greater efforts than the interpretation of speech (Sperber & Wilson, 1986). As a result, we tend to endorse rather than query the transitivizing nature of silence.

Filling the gap of silence is also prevalent in educational settings. The banking model of education does not embrace silence, for it aims at "depositing" knowledge into students' minds rather than "facilitating" students' reflective evaluation of knowledge claims. Although there are silent gaps in teachers' talks, lectures, power point presentations, and endless web pages, in general, these gaps are meaningless and have to be filled immediately in order not to interrupt the process of knowledge transmission. Teachers are meaningfully silent only when they are in the process of evaluating their students' abilities to "reproduce" the factual information and knowledge disseminated by them. From a Foucauldtian perspective, the silent teachers, like priests or psychotherapists, are able to exercise institutional power over the students because they are in the position of judging students' self-disclosure. At the same time, students can employ silence as a device for resisting knowledge transmission. This model denotes that speech making is the essence of teaching and learning; that is, if there is no speech either in written or verbal format, there is little or no learning/teaching.

To a large extent, this model of education reflects a particular cultural belief that the whole universe is knowable (Davies, 1992) and continuous expansion/refinement of the existing knowledge system can eventually attain a complete understanding of the universe (Rose, 2001). To Deborah Bird Rose (2001), such a progress-oriented theory of knowledge does not require a presumption that "silence must amount to an absence of knowledge; . . . but the moral ground of this theory depends on representing its own knowledge as the measure of knowledge, and representing as a universal good the idea that knowledge is becoming ever more complete. It thus argues forcibly against the concealment of knowledge, and renders plausible the idea that *silences in others signals an absence of knowledge*" (emphasis added) (p. 94). The pursuit of progress in the educational arena suggests that a linear progressive process of learning/teaching is the norm at both macro and micro levels. Hence, so-called Third World nations must make progress toward industrialization, advanced bureaucratization, and pluralistic democracy, as epitomized by developed nations (Welch, 1999). In a similar vein, teaching and learning in the classroom setting must observe a linear series of predetermined activities in order to attain predetermined curricular objectives pertaining to the progressive completion of the knowledge system.

Granted, recent professional teacher education programs have made significant efforts to reconstruct lecture-oriented teaching, and the emerging primacy of cooperative learning in mainstream teaching education programs clearly indicates teacher educators' commitment to promoting interactive teaching and learning. Still, speech making continues to function as the cornerstone of teaching and learning. Also, it is common to separate professional educational researchers and professional practitioners, despite the recent advocacy of "teacher-as-researcher." In accordance with such a division of labor, professional educational researchers are responsible for undertaking scientific research in order to build up a solid knowledge base of teaching and learning. In other words, educational researchers are the authorities and sources of pedagogical knowledge while educational practitioners are expected to consult with educational researchers and further observe a set of rules/rubrics formulated by educational researchers. Donald A. Schön (1983) points out that such dependence on scientific method reflects a "technical rationality" that dominates most teacher training programs. According to such technical rationality, teaching and learning are a linear series of pre-determined activities, which may include the use of silence when the use of silence can be proved to be fruitful for learning. To illustrate, M. E. Rowe's well-known study of wait-time includes the following findings:

1. The length of student response increased from a mean of seven words to a mean of 27 words.
2. The mean number of appropriate unsolicited responses increased from five to 17.
3. Mean failure to respond dropped from seven to one.
4. Mean incidence of evidence-inference statements increased from six to 14.
5. Average incidence of soliciting, structuring, and reacting moves increased from five to 32.
6. Number of speculative responses increased from a mean of two to a mean of seven.
7. Incidence of student-student comparison of data increased.
8. Frequency of student-initiated questions increased from a mean of one to a mean of four. (Rowe, 1974, pp. 221–22)

Based on the above findings, Rowe concludes that the use of silence—wait-time—can improve the quality of classroom interaction. It is apparent that Rowe's argument is based on the assumption that the quality of classroom interaction is determined by the quantity of interactions. Thus, the pedagogical purpose of silent wait-time is simply to entail verbal responses. While Rowe does attend to the number of speculative responses, it is clear that silent speculation cannot be observed and measured. Hence, the verbalization of students' speculation is the only measurable indicator of the quality of classroom interaction. Informed by Rowe's study, teachers learn to utilize silent wait-time in the process of teaching in order to provide essential temporal space for thinking and reflection. However, the current accountability movement is so outcome driven that many teachers are inclined to view silence as a mechanical device for soliciting observable and measurable responses in either verbal or written form. Hence, modern schooling may recognize the instrumental values of silence in facilitating more speech making; but silence as a pedagogical action may not be grounded in teachers' mindful reflections on teaching and learning.

In support of D. A. Schön's advocating teachers' engagement in "reflection-in-action," Robert Tremmel (1999) claims that Zen Buddhism as an alternative epistemological tradition to "technical rationality" sheds significant light on the possibility of reflective and mindful teaching. Robert Tremmel points out that the western cultural conception of "reflection" tends to emphasize "analysis and problem-solving." In contrast, Zen reflection does not aim at specific predetermined outcomes or search for desirable outcomes. Instead, Zen reflection embraces a mindful awareness of "here and now." To a large extent, the western conception of reflection relies upon speech/language in defining terms and concepts, formulating hypotheses, and evaluating outcomes in a very linear process. As language and speech are highly structured and regulated, one's undertaking speech acts can easily distract one's engagement in what Zen Buddhists view as mindful and reflective process. D. T. Suzuki (1959/1989) states: "Zen is not necessarily against words, but is well aware of the fact that they are always liable to detach themselves from realities and turn into conceptions. And this conceptualization is what Zen is against. . . . Zen insists on handling the thing itself and not an empty abstraction." From Suzuki's standpoint, the devaluation of words/speech in Zen Buddhism derives from the recognition of the limitation of language. Likewise, Indian yoga tradition also discredits verbalism and embraces silence. Accordingly, S. N. Ganguly (1968–69) argues that silence is "the limit of our world of description or language" and "silence is silence and completely different from any kind of language" (p. 200). In the same vein, Max Picard (1988) states:

> When language ceases, silence begins. But it does not begin BECAUSE language ceases. The absence of language simply makes the presence of Silence more apparent. Silence is an autonomous phenomenon. It is therefore not identical with the suspension of language. It is not merely the negative condition that sets in when the positive is removed; it is rather an independent whole, subsisting in and through itself. (p. 17)

On the one hand, the above perspectives are problematic because the search for the essence of silence can easily result in an infinite regress of definitions. On the other hand, these perspectives are helpful for recasting the silence as an inward spiritual state for reflective thinking. Silence, devoid of regulative linguistic structures, can be conducive for both teachers and students to raise awareness of "here and now."

Max Van Manen (1990) classifies three types of silence: literal silence, epistemological silence, and ontological silence. To Van Manen, literal silence refers to the absence of speaking. From Van Manen's perspective, because speech may not convey all of human thoughts, emotions, and actions, more speech does not necessarily generate better human communication. It follows that the pedagogical use of silence such as wait-time should not intend to create awkwardness or discomfort in order to solicit *more* prescribed or desirable verbal responses, as implied in M. E. Rowe's study of wait-time. On the contrary, absence of speaking can be invaluable to facilitate reflections on human communication. As discussed before, there is a lack of appreciation of silence in formal educational settings in most modern societies. In addition to the progress-oriented epistemological tradition, the desire or perceived need to make more speech reflects the capitalist economy, marked by mass production and mass consumption. The commodification of knowledge at the higher education level especially seduces or compels professional scholars and researchers to be "productive" in making speeches, an equivalence of making goods. Since parsimony of speech making is not the norm, "silence" appears to be an alienating idea and a rare practice in formal educational institutions. However, the flourishing of scholarly publications does not necessarily facilitate more mindful social and school reforms. Similarly, as the most eloquent and vocal teachers and students monopolize discursive practices in the group settings, cooperative learning and collaborative inquiry are bound to fail.

To redress the inadequacy of speech making at both individual and collective levels, it might be important for concerned educators to silently contemplate what has been left unsaid. The purpose of such contemplation does not aim at translating "silence" into "speech." Rather, it raises our awareness of the limitations of speech and the need to explore varied forms of communication. For instance, S. U. Philips (1985) calls our attention to "interaction through silence" in formal educational institutions. Such silent interaction can "incorporate all the situations in which the silent, nonverbal, physical, visual, and other signals override speech in interpreting the communicative behavior of the participant(s), although speech and other vocal signals may be present and need not be excluded from the interpretation of a given speech situation structured through silence" (Jaworski, 1993, p. 18). In highly structured educational institutions, teachers as well as students gradually acquire tacit knowledge in encoding and decoding silent interaction. Furthermore, they are fully aware of the clear demarcation between acceptable and unacceptable silent interaction even though the rules are rarely spelled out.

Many educational ethnographers further note that students' success in school is not solely determined by their acquisition of academic knowledge. Rather, students' success, to a large extent, depends upon when and how they display acceptable interaction competence in classroom settings. Such interaction competencies often constitute students' attitude toward learning. To illustrate, Perry Gilmore's study (1985) points out that academic tracking can be based on students' silent attitudes. He also notes that teachers and students all use silence to negotiate their power relationships. However, whereas teachers tend to exert and display power, students are more inclined to defy and claim power. In view of the significant impact of students' attitudes, reflective teachers must attend to and redress the asymmetric power relationship that exists in the silent interaction so they can listen with "the third ear" to what is often left unsaid (Reik, 1948). In short, it is not necessary to structure teaching solely through talk/speech and foster students' exclusive commitment to speech making. Furthermore, it is imprudent to "evaluate" students' learning according to their "verbal participation" in in-class learning activities. In contrast, it is important for educators to inquire into silence as "revelatory enactment" so that we do not compel students to "talk" for the sake of "talking" (Corcoran, 2000).

Van Manen (1990) defines epistemological silence as human beings' experiencing the ineffability of certain types of knowledge or skills in certain contexts. According to Van Manen, human experiences of ineffability can be individual- or group-based; i.e., individuals or groups may have limited or variegated linguistic competence depending upon the temporal contexts, subject matters, format of discourse, and institutional cultures. As the linear process of teaching and learning moves toward predetermined curricular goals/objectives, both students and teachers often accept temporal constraints of teaching and learning as given. Thus, teachers and students are reluctant to ponder over or inquire into what is ineffable within the particular temporal context. As a result, teachers and students conspire to keep the wait-time as short as possible. Such a rush to make a speech can easily construct a highly competitive social milieu to praise the talker and shame the listeners. Instead of promoting quick response as a demonstration of intellectual prowess that preys on silent students, concerned educators might want to endorse silent active listening or thinking as a legitimate and essential component of learning, especially in a group setting.

With respect to epistemological silence on subject matters, it should be noted that modern schooling does not include a critical self-examination of what Gregory Bateson (1972) calls "the frame" of the progress-oriented epistemological tradition that shapes curricular planning and daily teaching. According to Bateson (1972), the frame is "involved in the evaluation of the messages . . . as such the frame is metacommunicative" (p. 188). As "the frame" determines the legitimacy of knowledge claims, our ineffability on some phenomenon may indicate the inadequacy of "the frame" rather than an individual's intellectual inadequacy. Hence, the experience of epistemological silence on certain subject matters can be a teachable moment that invites us to explore alternative frames. Furthermore, epistemological silence can be related to our keen awareness of the limitations of language/speech. Gayatri C. Spivak (1987) points out: "The problem of human discourse is generally seen as articulating itself in the play of, in terms of, three shifting 'concepts': language, world, and consciousness. We know no world that is not organized as language, we operate with no other consciousness but one structured as a language—language that we cannot possess, for we are operated by those languages as well; language then, embraces the categories of world and consciousness even as it is determined by them" (pp. 77–78). Epistemological silence as the indicator of the breakdown of the interlocking triad (language, world, and consciousness) can raise our awareness of how these dynamic factors contribute to the process of knowledge construction.

According to Van Manen (1990), ontological silence indicates an awareness of "the realization of our fundamental predicament of always returning to silence—even or perhaps especially after the most enlightening speech, reading, or conversation" (p. 114). This type of silence is in-between content and discontent with discursive practices. Often, ontological silence is neither an invitation to make more speech nor an initiation to pursue absolute silence. Instead of sustaining the dichotomy of silence and speech, ontological silence indicates a need to attend to the dynamic interconnections between them. In an attempt to demystify the absolutized boundary of language, Yoru Wang (2001) applies a liminological approach to illumine Chan Buddhists' thoughts on the interplay of speech and silence. The liminological approach emphasizes "the relativization of any limits of language" (Wang, 2001, p. 83). In other words, the limits of language are two-sided, i.e., "the inadequacy of language runs the risk of never being sufficiently inadequate" (Blanchot, 1981, p. 129). Similarly, silence, defined as the absence of speech/language, is not so complete that we are not in need of speech. In challenging the absolute boundaries of speech and silence, Wang (2001) calls our attention to the Middle Way that "maintains a nirvanic dimension in the everyday world without presupposing a transcendental realm. By the same token, it pinpoints the insufficiency of conventional language without postulating any sacred language (whether a metalanguage or complete silence)" (p. 91). Wang (2001) points out that the Middle Way "is like a thread running through the Buddha's teaching, Mâdhyamika discourse, and Chan practice" (p. 89). The value of the Middle Way is based on its acknowledgment of the complementary interconnections and continuum between speech and silence. In other words, the Middle Way does not aim at silencing speech. Rather, it advocates for a nondualistic demystification of the perceived incommensurability between speech and silence. In adopting the Middle Way approach, concerned educators can be more attentive to what is beyond and beneath speech as well as what is in-between silence and speech. In the next section, I will further examine the practical viability of the Middle Way by exploring the merits and demerits of critically minded educators' attempts to reclaim silenced voices and to silence oppressive silences at both macro and micro levels.

Reclaiming Silenced Voices and Silencing Silence

As mentioned before, silencing as a disciplinary act reveals and sustains imbalanced power relationships between individuals and between groups. The state of silence signifies a state of oppression. In confronting cultural imperialism, Gloria Anzaldua (1987) pointedly exclaims that "The Anglo with the innocent face has yanked our tongue, thus sentencing colonized cultural beings to silenced culture. Drowned, we spit darkness. Fighting with our very shadow we are buried by silence" (p. 203). In view of the oppressive impacts of silencing, modern political theorists such as Hannah Arendt (1958), F. R. Dallmyr (1984), and Jürgen Habermas (1987) argue that making a speech is taking a political action formally and informally. Jürgen Habermas (1979) especially strives to articulate the "ideal speech act" as a means to the emancipation of the oppressed even though he is fully aware that speech can be systematically distorted to privilege some individuals or some groups over others. To silenced people, the desire and ability to speak out is a liberating process. For instance, bell hooks (1989) points out that "Moving from silence into speech is for the oppressed, the colonized, the exploited, and those who stand

and struggle side by side a gesture of defiance that heals, that makes new life and new growth possible" (p. 9). Henry Giroux and Peter McLaren (1986) also state that the minority students' voice "is the discursive means to make themselves 'heard' and to define themselves as active authors of their worlds" (p. 213). Reclaiming silenced voices thus has emerged as the central theme of the recent postmodern multicultural education movement. To many concerned educators, the reclaimed silenced voices are the liberatory voices that could redress historical injustice at the macro level. At the micro level, many educators also strive to establish an ideal discursive community in the classroom, where the "silenced" students can "speak out." Metaphorically, these educators are eager to silence silences in order to achieve human liberation. However, there are problems with endorsing silencing silences as the primary liberatory pedagogical practice.

First, educational efforts to reclaim silenced voices reflect the politics of identity in the late twentieth century. Academic and political discourse on marginalized groups' "struggle for recognition" tends to identify the marginalized groups as passive victims. The call for due recognition of marginalized people often embraces the belief that freedom of speech is an inalienable human right. Silencing silences thus emerges as a liberation movement to transform passive victims into active agents. To illustrate, Charles Taylor (1992) states: "Nonrecognition or misrecognition . . . can be a form of oppression, imprisoning someone in a false, distorted, reduced mode of being. Beyond simple lack of respect, it can inflict *a grievous wound,* saddling people with crippling self-hatred. Due recognition is not just a courtesy but a human need" (p. 25) (emphasis added). Thus, Taylor endorses "a politics of universalism, emphasizing the equal dignity of all citizens, and the content of this politics has been the equalization of rights and entitlements" (p. 37). In other words, the politics of due recognition is to ensure that the wounded are equal to the members of the dominant groups, who are neither wounded nor silenced. Notwithstanding Taylor's noble attempt to equalize human rights and entitlement, I agree with Wendy Brown (1995) that the identification of a marginalized minority as "a wound" is disturbing because such "wounded attachments" can easily reduce the victims to objects of oppression. Also, while various forms of public silencing have deprived silenced people of their right to public speech, it is misleading to assume that silenced people are unable to protest and resist silencing. The identification of the state of silence as a state of absolute oppression fails to recognize that the silenced can be complicit in the cultural practice of their silences (Smith, 1987). Granted, silenced people's complicity in social silence can be a coping strategy in many circumstances, but the silenced people's complicity as the last resort certainly does not justify the act of public silencing. Nevertheless, recognition of possible complicity acknowledges the silenced people's human agency. Without recognizing the silenced people's agency in resistance and complicity, a liberating effort to reclaim silenced voices may appear to be groundless. After all, a true liberation should mean that the silenced people are able speak for themselves, as suggested by Paulo Freire.

Furthermore, it should be noted that members of dominant groups could imprison themselves in "a false, distorted, reduced mode of being," too. In examining women's being silenced in most cultures, Susan Gal (1990) finds that while the silenced women may be powerless in the public domain, they are able to develop alternative communicative skills, such as attentiveness and responsiveness to others in conversation. She further points out, "the fact that social silence has neglected women makes women of the past and other cultures seem silent, when in fact the silence is that of current western scholarship" (Gal, 1990, p. 426). In other words, the silencers cannot escape the pervasive impact of silencing "the others" because they must subject themselves to the rules that justify the act of oppressive silencing. In consequence, the silencers deprive themselves of the right to listen to or acquire the capacities of speaking in different voices. Hence, if it is oppressive to force the silenced to endure oppressive silence, it is equally oppressive for the oppressors to be committed to the act of silencing.

Speech as the inalienable human right does not necessarily entail the right of being listened to. To facilitate an empathetic listening, one must attend to the contexts in which forced silences occur. Edward Said (1994) expounded that one must develop an exilic intellectuals' ability to "see things not simply as they are, but as they have come to be that way. Look at situations as contingent, not as inevitable, look at them as the result of a series of historical choices made by men and women, as facts of society made by human beings" (p. 60). To develop the ability to see things "as they have come to be that way," one must listen to silences. In *Articulate Silence,* King-Kok Cheung (1993), makes concerted efforts to demystify the absolute power of silencing by explicating how silences such as voiceless gestures, textual ellipses, and authorial hesitations, are embedded in three second-generation Asian American women: Hisaye Yamamoto, Maxine Hong Kingston, and Joy Kogawa. Their silences not only interrogate the authorities but also shed light on the complicated yet articulate nature of silences. It follows that a genuine effort to reclaim the silenced voices must acknowledge that the silenced voices are not the absence of speech. Otherwise, the silenced people's reclaiming their silenced voices can simply function as a reassurance of the oppressive power of the dominant group. A truly liberating pedagogy must be based on a conjoint effort to listen to the silences and to reclaim the silenced voices. This approach is not based on a sequential logic; i.e., listening to silences first and reclaiming the silenced voices later. Rather, it calls our attention to interconnections between speech and silence. After all, if the oppressors' right to speech does not prevent their dehumanization, it is doubtful that the silenced people's speech making can immunize human societies from varied forms of oppression. Listening to the silences can facilitate a more in-depth understanding of silenced people's agency in coping with and in negotiating with oppression.

It should be noted that silenced people's reclaiming of their voices often relies upon their mastery of the dominant groups' languages. A marginalized group's development of dexterity in the dominant group's rhetoric and logical devices can be indispensable for the political actions that demand equality and justice. The women's movement and the civil rights movement in the United States, to a large extent, simultaneously embrace and discredit the fundamental principles of liberalism, such as equality and justice. Although bell hooks (1996) recognizes the liberating force of moving from silence to speech, she also notes that many African Americans view "English" as the "oppressor's language which has the potential to disempower those of us who are just learning to speak, who are just learning to claim language as a place where we make ourselves subject." Audre Lorde (1984) echoes bell hooks's concern: "Certainly for Black women our struggle has not been to emerge from silence to speech but to change the nature and direction of our speech. To make a speech that compels listeners, one that is heard" (p. 124). However, is it speech that compels listeners? Is it the receptive listener who makes the speech compelling or is it the changing cultural and political climate that compels listeners?

In view of the intertwined relationship among speech, speakers, listeners, and the social milieu, it is clear that silencing silences alone cannot be an effective political action to end oppression. After all, it is doubtful that the oppressors must "hear" the silenced people's compelling speech in order to be aware of their perils. It is quite uncertain that the dominant will surrender their privileges upon listening to the reclaimed silenced voices. In fact, it is more likely that the dominant groups will desire to enhance and preserve the privileges that have led to the oppressive silencing in the first place. Thus, it is not surprising that silenced people often face the threat of exile or the demand of their going back to where they came from when they make efforts to reclaim their silenced voices. For instance, in his efforts to pursue peace in his homeland, the Vietnamese monk Thich Nhat Hanh found it necessary to travel to the United States. In 1968, he delivered a speech in a wealthy Christian church in a St. Louis suburb. Despite his plea for compassion, an audience confronted him with scornful query: "If you care so much about your people, Mr. Hanh, why are you here? If you care so much for the people who are wounded, why don't you spend your time with them?" After a deep moment of silence, Nhat Hanh responded, "If you want the tree to grow, it won't help to water the leaves. You have to water the roots. Many of the roots of the war are here, in your country. To help the people who are to be bombed, to try to protect them from this suffering, I have to come here" (Forest, 1987, p. 103). Clearly, to make a compelling speech to power is not an easy task as the dominant group can simply refuse to listen and even demand the banishment of the silenced people who dare to speak. Edward Said (1994) comments: "Speaking the truth to power is not Panglossian idealism: it is carefully weighing the alternatives, picking the right one, and then intelligently representing it where it can do the most good and cause the right change" (p. 102). However, is it fair to put an undue burden on the silenced people to make compelling speeches in order to shape the zeitgeist for social reform movements?

In particular, it should be noted that efforts to reclaim silenced voices often result in full-blown recognition of the silenced people's vanishing cultures rather than in acknowledgment and commitment to the distribution of economic resources, which are indispensable for their "capabilities to function" in the societies, as suggested by Amartya Sen (1985). Consequently, while reclaiming silences voices can raise our awareness of cultural diversity, we also justify the dominant group's ignorance and the resultant unjust distribution of material resources. It is not surprising that the Marxist theory of capitalist exploitation remains insightful yet ineffective in redressing economic inequality. To a large extent, it is not the Marxists who fail to make compelling speech. Rather, it is the dominant group's unwillingness to relinquish their unfair share of economic resources. In view of the dehumanizing effects of inequality on dominant groups, concerned educators must attend to facilitating the dominant groups' commitment to unpacking their presumably "invisible privileges" at the macro level, as suggested by Peggy McIntosh (1989). In other words, making eloquent or compelling speech alone is not the key to silencing the oppressive silences. Rather, liberation demands a reflective ethical commitment to justice and equality.

Similarly, while it is encouraging that there has been a burgeoning of book series that document, interpret, and disseminate indigenous local knowledge systems, the demand for "differences" has not resulted in establishing inclusive and extensive social justice. To Ladi Semali and Joe Kincheloe (2000), the editors of the book series: Indigenous Knowledge and Schooling, it is essential and feasible to "use indigenous knowledge to counter Western science's destruction of the earth. Indigenous knowledge can facilitate this ambitious twenty-first century project because of its tendency to focus on relationships of human beings to both one another and to their ecosystem." While the naming of "indigenous knowledge" reveals an effort to revitalize the marginalized or even "disappearing" cultural traditions, it also suggests that we ought to preserve not-yet-contaminated indigenous knowledge because of its pragmatic utility in solving the social ills of the postmodern and postindustrial societies. Trinh Minh-ha (1989) points out that "the Third World representative which the modern sophisticated public ideally seeks is the *unspoiled* African, Asian, or Native American, who remains more preoccupied with her/his image of the *real* native—the *truly different*—than with issues of hegemony, racism, feminism, and social change" (p. 88) (emphasis original).

Unfortunately, such "differences" can be easily transformed into the form of commodity in advanced capitalism. Patricia Hill Collins (2000) further argues, "the difference to be commodified is an authentic, essential difference long associated with group differences of race, ethnicity, gender, economic class, and sexuality" (p. 32). The cult for authenticity or even purity of the marginalized voices not only fossilizes the marginalized groups' cultures but also prescribes a specific role for the marginalized groups—victims of the oppressive cultural hegemony rather than active agents who are capable of undertaking cultural transformation to counter hegemonic power. As the essentialization of silenced voices leads consumers to quest for specific voices in terms of formats and contents, reclaiming silenced voices inevitably leads to the silencing of unmarketable voices at the macro level. In short, although the commodification of marginalized and silenced voices and the consumption of otherness certainly contribute to the diversification of scholarly discourses, they also distract needed attentions from the imbalanced power relationships among various groups in the political and economic dimensions.

Silencing silences as a primary pedagogical and political action appears to reaffirm the primacy of speech and perpetuate the dominant groups' speech as the norm at the macro level. In classroom settings, it is common for teachers to devalue silences and promote speech making. Teachers often enlist "participation" as an evaluation criterion. But, they do not recognize "silent active listening" as a legitimate form of participation. As teachers attend to students' speech making, they frequently fail to acknowledge the significance of the silent interactions between teachers and students that reveal human desires, interests, and power relationships. Consequently, although teachers are able to compel students to engage in verbal participation in classroom settings, they are unlikely to hear and listen to students' inner voices that do not meet their expectations. In addition to the above parallels between silencing silences at macro and micro levels, it is important to undertake a further inquiry into the moral condemnation of silencing and the political imperatives of silencing silences in the classroom.

Advocates of critical pedagogy are fully aware of the intricate connections between politics and education. In *A Pedagogy for Liberation,* Paulo Freire claims:

> There is a great discovery, education is politics! When a teacher discovers that he or she is a politician, too, the teacher has to ask, What kind of politics am I doing in the classroom? That is, in favor of whom am I being a teacher? The teacher works in favor of something and against something. Because of that, he or she will have another great question, How to be consistent in my teaching practice with my political choice? (Shor & Freire, 1987, p. 46)

Although politics and education are inseparable, it is problematic to assume that teachers can transform their platform into a soapbox without addressing imbalanced power relationships in the formal educational setting. Also, the oppositional approach, to a large extent, oversimplifies the complex nature of varied forms of political or economic oppression. As a result, transformative critical pedagogy can be reduced to moral condemnation of the act of silencing in classroom settings. More specifically, many educators like Jacqui Alexander and Chandra Mohanty (1997) believe that "education was a key strategy of decolonization, rather than merely a path toward mainstream credentials and upward mobility" (p. xviii). Accordingly, education should aim at redressing the exclusion of marginalized cultures from the formal curriculum. In addition to developing critiques of the established canon that endorses western cultural hegemony, there are deliberate efforts to delineate the connections between the presumably universal disciplines, such as science and mathematics, and varied marginalized cultures. Often, such a critical inclusive approach entails a moral condemnation of the act of silencing and sanctions an oppositional mode of thinking as a revolutionary praxis. As discussed before, although the political imperative of silencing silences intends to generate empathy in order to heal "the wound," the perpetual perception of the victimhood of the silenced does not acknowledge the agency of the silenced and the dehumanization of the silencers. Moreover, it does not encourage members of the dominant group to assume moral responsibility for facilitating social transformation. Instead, moral condemnation of silencing tends to entrap students in guilt or resentment.

Wendy Brown (1995) asked: "Could we learn to contest domination with the strength of an alternative vision of collective life, rather than through moral reproach?" (p. 47). For instance, in exploring alternative visions of collective life, the advocacy of bilingual education cannot focus solely on the linguistic and cultural minority groups' collective rights—as if the linguistic and cultural majority groups are entitled or even destined to be "monolingual." Rather, it is important to recognize all students' educational rights to be bilingual or multilingual. In *The Violence of Language*, J. J. Lecercle (1991) takes note of the incomplete nature of any given language system. According to Lecercle, each given language system has well-defined rules of grammar, syntax, and semantics. While strict observance of rules can ensure effective communication, abandonment of the rules does not necessarily impede human communication because each language system contains "the remainder" that is beyond the regulation of the linguistic rules. In other words, the fundamental rule of "the remainder" is an entitlement or freedom to ignore all the linguistic rules. Similarly, it should be noted that no legal or cultural system is so complete that no amendments or complementary human actions are allowed or needed. Just as there are no "remainderless" linguistic, legal, cultural, and identity systems, concerned educators must be aware that silencing silences is not the consummation of liberation. On the contrary, it is important to attend to "the remainder"—what is beneath silences and beyond silencing silences. To illustrate, Sharon E. Sutton's (1996) inquiry into how material conditions shape students' worldviews and identities sheds light on the non-linguistic contributing factors of successful educational and social reforms. Similarly, David W. Orr (1994) reminds us:

> The curriculum embedded in any building instructs as fully and as powerfully as any course taught in it. . . . There is often a miscalibration between the lesson of inter-connectedness when it is taught in classes and the way a building, campus, or school actually functions. . . . When the pedagogical abstractions, words, and whole courses do not fit the way the buildings and landscape constituting the academic campus in fact work, they (students) learn that hope is just wishful thinking or worse, rank hy-pocrisy. (pp. 140, 141, 147)

Instead of focusing on making more speech to condemn the dominant ideology, Orr (1994) initiates and implements a project to design a building that promotes "ecological competence and mindfulness" (p. 141). Orr's insight into the silent pedagogy does not call for an elimination of vocal pedagogy. It simply indicates that socially responsive pedagogy must go beyond silencing silences.

All in all, silence and speech are the inseparable foundations of human communication. However, the dichotomization of silence and speech misleads us to devalue silence and privilege speech. My affirmation of the pedagogical merits of silences does not aim at "silencing" speech. Rather, I call for recognition of the need to dismantle this false dichotomy and to develop a pedagogical understanding of silences.

References

Alexander, M. J. & Mohanty, C. T. (1997). *Feminist genealogies, colonial legacies, democratic future*. New York: Routledge.

Anzaldua. G. (1987). *Borderlands: The new Mestiza*. San Francisco: Spinsters/Aunt Lute.

Arendt, H. (1958). *The human condition*. Chicago: University of Chicago Press.

Bateson, G. (1972). *Steps to an ecology of the mind*. New York: Ballantine.

Blanchot, M. (1981). *The gaze of Orpheus and other literacy essays*. Barrytown, NY: Station Hill Press.

Brown, W. (1995). Wounded attachments: Late modern oppositional political formations. In J. Rajchman (Ed.), *The identity in question* (pp. 199–228). New York: Routledge.

Cheung, K. (1993). *Articulate silences: Hisaye Yamoto, Maxine Hong Kinston, Joy Kogawa*. Ithaca, NY and London: Cornell University Press.

Collins, P. H. (2000). What's going on? Black feminist thought and the politics of postmodernism. In E. A. St. Pierre & W. S. Pillow (Eds.), *Working the ruins: Feminist poststructural theory and methods in education* (pp. 27–40). New York: Routledge.

Cook, J. J. (1964). Silence in psychotherapy. *Journal of Counseling Psychology, 11*(1), 42–46.

Corcoran, P. (2000). Silence. In P. Corcoran and V. Spender (Eds.), *Disclosures* (pp. 172–201). Aldershot: Ashgate.

Dallmayr, F. R. (1984). *Language and politics: Why does language matter to political philosophy?* Notre Dame: University of Notre Dame Press.

Dauenhauer, B. P. (1980). *Silence: The phenomenon and its ontological significance*. Bloomington: Indiana University Press.

Davies, P. (1992). *The mind of God: The scientific basis for a rational world*. New York: Simon & Schuster.

Dumont, R. V. Jr. (1972). Learning English and how to be silent: Studies in Sioux and Cherokee classrooms. In C. B. Cazden, V. P. John & D. Hymes (Eds.), *Functions of language in the classroom* (pp. 370–394). Prospect Heights, IL: Waveland Press.

Enninger, W. (1987). What interactants do with non-talk across cultures. In K. Knapp, W. Enninger, & A. Knapp-Potthoff (Eds.), *Analyzing intercultural communication* (pp. 269–302). Berlin: Mouton de Gruyter.

Forest, J. (1987). Nhat Hanh: Seeing with the eyes of compassion. In *Thich Nhat Hanh: The miracle of mindfulness* (M. Ho, Trans.). Boston: Beacon Press.

Freire, P. (1970). *Pedagogy of the oppressed* (M. Bergman Ramos, Trans.). New York: Continuum.

Gal, S. (1990). Speech and silence: The problematics of research on language and gender. In M. di Leonardo (Ed.), *Gender at the crossroads of knowledge*. Berkley, CA: University of California Press.

Ganguly, S. N. (1968–69). Culture, communication, and silence. *Philosophy and Phenomenological Research*, 29, 200.

Gilmore, P. (1985). *Silence and sulking: Emotional display in the classroom*. In D. Tannen & M. Saville-Troike (Eds.), *Perspectives on silence*. Norwood, NJ: Ablex.

Giroux, H. A. & P. McLaren (1986). Teacher education and the politics of engagement: The case for democratic schooling. *Harvard Educational Review* 56(3), 213–238.

Greene, A. B. (1940). *The philosophy of silence*. New York: Richard R. Smith.

Habermas, J. (1979). *Communication and the Evolution of Society* (T. McCarthy, Trans.). Boston: Beacon Press.

Habermas, J. (1987). *Moral consciousness and communicative action* (C. Lenhardt and S. W. Nicholsen, Trans.). Cambridge: M.I.T Press.

hooks, b. (1989). *Taking back: Thinking feminist, thinking black*. Boston: South End Press.

hooks, b. (1996). *Teaching to transgress*. New York: Routledge.

Houston, M. & Kramarae, C. (1991). Speaking from silence: Methods of silencing and of resistance. *Discourse and Society* 2(4), 387–99.

Jaworski, A. (1993). *The power of silence: Social and pragmatic perspectives*. Newbury Park: SAGE Publications.

John, V. P. (1972). Styles of learning, styles of teaching: Reflections on the education of Navajo children. In C. B. Cazden, V. P. John, & D. Hymes (Eds.), *Functions of language in the classroom* (pp. 331–43). Prospect Heights, IL: Waveland Press.

Kurzon, D. (1998). *Discourse of silence*. Amsterdam/Philadelphia: John Benjamins Publishing Company.

Lazreg, M. (1994). *The eloquence of silence: Algerian women in question*. New York: Routledge.

Lecercle, J. J. (1991). *The violence of language*. London: Routledge.

Lorde, A. (1984). *Sister outsider*. Trumansburg, NY: Crossing Press.

McIntosh, P. (1989, July/August). White privilege: Unpacking the invisible knapsack. *Peace and Freedom*, 10–12.

Orr, D. W. (1994). Reassembling the pieces. In S. Glazer (Ed.), *The heart of learning: Spirituality in education* (pp. 139–150). New York: Penguin Putnam, Inc.

Philips, S. U. (1985). Interaction structured through talk and interaction structured through silence. In D. Tannen & M. Saville-Troike (Eds.), *Perspectives on silence* (pp. 205–13). Norwood, NJ: Ablex.

Picard, M. (1988). *The world of silence*. Washington, DC: Regnery Gateway.

Reik, T. (1948). *Listening with the third ear: The inner experience of a psychoanalyst.* New York: Farrar.

Rose, D. B. (2001). The silence and power of Women. In D. B. Rose (Ed.), *Words and silences: Aboriginal women, politics and land* (pp. 92–116). Crows Nest, Australia: Allen & Unwin.

Rowe, M. B. (1974). Pausing phenomena: Influence on the quality of instruction. *Journal of Psycholinguistic Research, 2(2),* 203–24.

Said, E. (1994). *Representations of the Intellectual.* New York: Vintage Books.

Schön, D. A. (1983). *The reflective practitioner: How professionals think in action.* New York: Basic Books.

Semali, L. & J. Kincheloe. (2000). Series editors' foreword. In R. Sambull Mosha (Ed.), *The Heartbeat of indigenous Africa: A study of the chagga educational system* (pp. ix–xvi). New York: Garland Publishing Inc.

Sen, A. (1985). *Commodities and capabilities.* New York: North-Hollond.

Shor, I., & P. Freire (1987). *A pedagogy for liberation: Dialogues on transforming education.* South Hadley, MA: Bergin and Garvey.

Smith, D. E. (1987). *The everyday world as problematic.* Milton Keynes, UK: Open University Press.

Sperber, D. & D. Wilson. (1978). *Relevance: Communication and cognition.* Oxford: Blackwell.

Spivak, G. (1987). *In other worlds: Essays in culture and politics.* New York: Methuen.

Sutton, S. E. (1996). *Weaving a tapestry of resistance: The place, power, and poetry of a sustainable society.* London: Bergin & Garvey.

Suzuki, D. T. (1989). *Zen and Japanese culture.* Princeton: Princeton University Press. (Original work published in 1859)

Taylor, C. (1992). *Multiculturalism and the politics of recognition.* Princeton: Princeton University Press.

Tremmel, R. (1999). Zen and the art of reflective practice in teacher education. In E. Mintz & J. T. Yun (Eds.). *The complex world of teaching: Perspectives from theory and practice* (pp. 87–110). Cambridge: Harvard University Press.

Trinh, M. (1989). *Woman, native, other: Writing postcoloniality and feminism.* Bloomington: Indiana University.

Van Manen, M. (1990). Researching lived experience: Human science for an action sensitive pedagogy. Albany: State University of New York Press.

Wang, Y. (2001). Liberating oneself from the absolutized boundary of language: A liminological approach to the interplay of speech and silence in Chan Buddhism. *Philosophy East and West,* 51(1), 83–99.

Weis, L., & M. Fine. (Eds.). (1993). *Beyond silenced voices: Class, race, and gender in United States schools.* Albany: State University of New York Press.

Welch, A. (1999). The triumph of technocracy or the collapse of certainty? Modernity, postmodernity, and postcolonialism in comparative education. In R. F. Arnove and C. A. Torres (Eds.), *Comparative education: The dialectic of the global and the local* (pp. 25–49). New York: Rowman & Littlefield Publishers.

Wilmer, H. A. (2000). *Quest for silence.* Am Klosterplatz, Switzerland: Daimon Verlag.

Zimmerman, M., & P. Rojas. (1998). *Voices from the silence: Guatemalan literature of resistance.* Athens: Ohio University Center for International Studies.

PART III

Moral and Philosophical Dimensions of Dialogue

Jim Garrison

Ameliorating Violence in Dialogues Across Differences: The Role of Eros and Lógos

My essay locates a primary source of troubling speech and disturbing silence in the sources of western philosophy and its tendency to reduce all difference to the sameness of its metaphysical and logical categories, concepts, and canons of identity construction. In my state (Virginia), for example, we reduce all differences to the same standards of learning (SOLs). I rely on Emmanuel Levinas and Jacques Derrida who provide compelling evidence that any approach to "the other" involving western discourse practices, including democratic discourse, is violent because of their reliance on western philosophy. Actually, I believe any linguistic form is violent simply because any structure, linguistic or otherwise, excludes what cannot satisfy its demands. Nonetheless, it is impossible to live without structure.

Violence in democratic dialogues across differences is inevitable simply because violence in all dialogues, or any other structured situation, is inevitable. For instance, The First Amendment right to freedom of speech seems crucial in structuring open democratic dialogues, yet it often excludes and oppresses those not empowered to speak. Nonetheless, we should seek to ameliorate violence wherever we find it. I propose a passionate ambivalence wherein we learn to live with ideas, emotions, and actions and their accompanying cognitive uncertainties. We must resist the notion we may ever know, recognize, or realize "the other" with absolute certainty, nor can we complete the quest for certainty backwards by proving the other is unknowable, unrecognizable, or unrealizable. We must learn to live creatively with the paradox. Passionate ambivalence in the pursuit of social amelioration calls for a cautious compassion that exercises moral imagination and perception in the attempt to concede the unique singularity of "the other" by refusing to reduce otherness and difference to the sameness of our self-identity. I will exercise passionate ambivalence in my conclusion when I criticize the limits of the discourse practices of political liberalism even as I defend its accomplishments.

There is a curious cognitive bias in discourse about the dangers of discourse. Because our primary relation to others is a cognitive knowing relation, I want to de-center the current conversation about alterity. Eventually, I associate passionate ambivalence and compassionate meliorism with eros (i.e., passionate desire). Emphasizing eros will not allow us to escape the violence of western (or eastern) thought, but it may allow us to practice intelligent violence against violence.

A life form is a biological structure. All living creatures live by consuming living creatures; being a vegetarian does not excuse you from the violence of participating in life's necessities, though it may ameliorate it. We should not renounce life because it is sometimes violent, nor should we renounce discourse because it is troubling or despair at silence, though it is often disturbing. Where there is the greatest danger in life, there also is the greatest possibility for creative growth.

Indoctrination, Education, and the Search for Sites of Compelling Critique

For any culture into which they are born, infants are initially "the other." All those who have taken the linguistic turn agree human beings are not born with minds or selves, much less free will or rationality; minds are achievements not endowments. Infants are not born with cultural meanings, values, and so on, and they only acquire them by participating in the discourse practices of their culture. Three of the most prominent philosophers of the twentieth century, John Dewey, Ludwig Wittgenstein, and Martin Heidegger, affirm such a stance. So do Levinas and Derrida, who acknowledge Heidegger's influence.

Each society imposes cultural structures (e.g., meanings, truths, and values) on its newborn. Schooling institutionalizes this process consciously, intentionally, and deliberately. Relying on Wittgenstein, C. J. B. Macmillan (1983) shows indoctrination is inevitable.[1] The basic argument is simple. According to Wittgenstein (1972), the linguistic propositions constituting an individual's world are precritical: "For how can a child immediately doubt what others are imparting to him? That could only mean that he was incapable of learning certain language games" (p. 283). Wittgenstein further observes, "The child learns by believing the adult. Doubt comes after belief" (p. 160). You cannot doubt a language game until you acquire one that plays the doubting game. Similar arguments work for other founding beliefs. Educators should come to terms with the inevitability of indoctrination. Some devotees of decontextualized rationality concede that indoctrination into rational world pictures is necessary, but they quickly add it is redeemable later by reasons.[2] Those indoctrinated in Christian communities prefer the redeemer. Of course, any successful indoctrination into a system of verification is subsequently self-justifiable. Some, like Derrida, find the entirety of western metaphysics or ontotheology equally violent, so they declare:

> My central question is: from what site or non-site (non-lieu) can philosophy as such appear to itself as other than itself, so that it can interrogate and reflect upon itself in an original manner? Such a non-site or alterity would be radically irreducible to philosophy. But the problem is that such a non-site cannot be defined or situated by means of philosophical language. (quoted in Kearney, 1984, p. 108)

Unfortunately, those indoctrinated in western philosophical thought, or any other form of life, structure, and so forth can never fully escape it. There are no neutral matrices allowing us to escape our cultural inheritance, although the dominant discourse of modern liberalism assumes there are. Innate reason and free will, decontextualized in some neutral mental realm outside space, time, and causation much less cultural practices, are leading liberal examples. Rejecting such utopian (literally, "not a place") sites, Derrida only seeks well-placed positions that allow critical latitude within the inescapable context of our indoctrination into some or another historically entrenched sociolinguistic practice. We will return to Derrida later when we examine his critique of Levinas.

Levinas on the Logos, Totality, and Infinity: The Violent Reduction of the "Other" to the Same

The etymology of the ancient Greek word *logos* (λογοζ) meaning "a discourse," "a dialogue," or "a speech," is important for the investigations of Levinas and Derrida. Indeed, any attempt at a fundamental understanding of speech in education must start here. We may trace the *logos* back to "the word" (λεγειυ) meaning "to tell." This is the sense we find at John 1:1 of the Bible, "In the beginning was the word [λογοζ] and the word was with God." John's story is perhaps the greatest ever told in the West. The contemporary rhetoric of the religious right regarding prayer and morality in the schools remains influential because it participates in the *logos* of Christian ontotheology.

The ancient violence of the western *logos* as dialogue is entrenched in the modern discourse practices of democratic liberalism that Levinas and Derrida deconstruct. Rational democracy, including communicative democracy, repeatedly reduces "the other" to the same logical categories, identities, etc. of the perceived normal, dutiful citizen. Although it is a form of violence for many, we should not forget democracy's achievements even as we fear its failures. As a form of violence, it still often stands against far worse forms, as the twentieth century amply proved.

It is a great mistake to believe we have achieved democracy when we have only begun the pursuit. As an institution, pluralistic democracy remains open to improvement and renewal in ways totalitarian forms of social life do not. Levinas (1961/1995) reveals the violence concealed in the western philosophy of the *logos*.

Western philosophy was born of the *logos* as telling the one true account of the essence (*eidos*) of some substance (*ousia*) that is the *telos* of some developmental process from origin or foundation (*archia*) to its perfection (*entelecheia*). Usually the *eidos, telos, entelecheia,* and *ousia* are indistinguishable. Supposedly, "normal" acorns grow up to become giant oak trees because that is their essence, substance, and perfect telos or *entelecheia*. Likewise, "normal" children grow up to become rational and God fearing adults as certified by test scores and disciplinary records. One size fits all; those who grow up different from the norm are deviant and, hence, defective. Because the *logos* assumes there is only one true discourse, it excludes all others. All these terms (*eidos, ousia, archia, entelecheia*) are associated with the metaphysics of substance, or what Derrida, following Heidegger, calls "the metaphysics of presence," and Levinas calls "ontology." This metaphysics, conjoined with the *logos,* has controlled western thought for over twenty-five hundred years, and subtly but pervasively influences how we think today about dialogue, schools, and difference.

Levinas locates the violence in the exclusivity of the rational *logos* (what Derrida calls logocentrism or phallocentrism) that always strives to reduce the "Other" to the "same" (the norm, the one true essence).[3] This is the logic of what he calls "ontology," which yields what he terms "totality." Nothing, no difference or alterity, escapes totalization. Western philosophy for Levinas has been almost entirely an ontology that attempts to achieve "a reduction of the other to the same by interposition of a middle and [supposedly] neutral term" (1961/1995, p. 43). The neutral mediator might be the ideal of "truth" common to all, the Absolute at the end of history in Hegel and Marx, innate rationality and freedom (including the free market) in liberalism, or God.

The rhetoric of supposedly value neutral standards and norm-referenced tests reduce many potential classroom dialogues to a concealed soliloquy of the same. Such mediators are all functions of "sovereign reason" that knows only itself because "nothing other limits it" (p. 43). Totalitarian reason reduces anything or anyone to the rule of its categories and concepts. Those who do not conform are condemned and expelled from the conversation. Dangerous discourse never arises because it finds no space not configured by the principles and identities defined by the *logos*. In western metaphysics, reason has no "Other" except error, or, in ontotheology, fallenness from grace into evil.

Ontology for Levinas is a philosophy of power and injustice (see p. 46). Here, the relation to the "Other" is that of the spectator at a safe, non-contaminating theoretical (from *theoreian*, a spectator from above) distance. It assumes our primary relation to "Other" is the knowing relation that reduces the other to the sameness of its own categories and purposes; therein resides the violence. Many teachers think they know their students because they know their grades and test scores. They do not think they need to understand their personalities, home life, or desires. We find the same thing in the theoretical orientation of the social sciences employed in education. Levinas finds that in the history of philosophy conflicts between the same and the Other are resolved by theoretically reducing the Other to the same (see p. 47). Megan Boler (this volume) shows how the marginalized are especially vulnerable to such hostilities. State educational technocrats reduce all difference and diversity to the same standards as measured by normalized tests, while punishing those outside the norms. Those who assume they can create safe spaces to sustain dialogues across difference in technocratic institutions must ignore the terrible asymmetries and inequalities of power perpetuated by technocratic rationality and its technologies. These are the people unwilling to move beyond issues of inclusiveness to issues of representation, ideology, identity construction, relational positionality, and authority in classrooms, schools, and communities.

Levinas contrasts what he calls "metaphysics" with ontology where we move from what he calls "need" to "desire." "Ordinarily, we assume need is the basis of desire and it gives rise to possessiveness. The ontological Eros seeks to possess the "Other" to satisfy its need. Possession is how the Other is most often reduced to the same. In possessive relations with the "Other," "Their *alterity* is . . . reabsorbed into my own identity as a . . . possessor" (p. 33). The needs of hunger, thirst, and sexuality frequently satisfy themselves in the kind of possession that strives to eradicate otherness, which results in violence and even cruelty (the conscious enjoyment of violence).

By contrast, the metaphysical desire abandons all hope of returning to itself. It is desire for the absolutely "Other." For Levinas, this Desire yields infinite transcendence because "the infinite is the absolutely other" (p. 49). Levinas believes no idea we may form is ever adequate to the absolute infinite other. Others "are not individuals of a common concept" instead, they appear as strangers who disturb my comfort because they are those over whom "I have no *power*" (p. 39). Levinas calls the presentation of the other that exceeds my own self-concept "face" (p. 50). Ontology satisfies our needs by drawing the "Other" into our selves; it cannot satisfy the eros for growth. Levinas distinguishes between ipsiety as self-sameness and perfect self-identity. We may remain qualitatively the same, though our identity may alter because we have become a quantitatively bigger version of our selves. Meanwhile, metaphysical desire draws us out toward the "Other" over whom we supposedly have no power.

The success of dialogues across difference depends less on ideas and more on attitudes of desire, imagination, possibilities, perceptions, risk, and vulnerability.

Most of the discourse on dialogues across differences assumes our primary relation to "Others" is a knowing relation. Almost everything I read about discourse, voice, silence, and difference constrains itself to the cognitive dimension. Actually, our relations to "Others" are more often aesthetic, ethical, embodied, affective, or even erotic. I want to concentrate on the erotic relation as a component in many successful dialogues across difference by emphasizing what Thomas M. Alexander (1993) calls the human eros, that is, the passionate desire to live a life of expanding meaning and value. Eros may satisfy itself by simply possessing or consuming its objects (food, water, the labor of slaves). The human eros, however, satisfies itself only when the "Other" draws us beyond our selves; for instance, when we listen carefully to what they are saying. Genuinely satisfying the human eros requires growing in such a way that we can never return to our former selves. That is because our transaction with those different from ourselves transforms our identity. Only the "Other" has the vocabulary, meanings, plot lines, grammar, truths, possibilities, and the like, we need to retell the story of our life; we need the "Other" if we are to be born again. Satisfying the human eros requires metaphysical Desire as Levinas describes it, for only "Others" different from our selves can provoke the creation of meanings and values beyond our culture's prescriptions.

To pursue the human eros, however, involves risk and vulnerability; therefore, it is dangerous especially to those whose eros is constrained and oppressed. Nonetheless, there is no growth without risk and vulnerability. Often, instead of attempting to construct safe spaces in their classroom, it would be better if teachers sought to grow in relationship with their students by rendering themselves vulnerable and at risk without necessarily requiring their students do the same. Sometimes it is best if we strive to become the change we wish to see in the world rather than demand that the world (and "Others" in it) change according to our demands. Teachers who teach this way will experience more difficulty as their personal identity evolves (and even fragments), but they are also the ones most likely to ameliorate the dangers of democratic dialogue across difference and collaboratively create the safest, though not sterile, educational communities. There is a kind of teaching that satisfies the teaching eros for self-expression by connecting with students and helping them grow. Vulnerability and risk open us up to growth, but people also get seriously hurt that way. No one grows who would remain secure, no one grows without loss, and some will be slain. When we prune plants for their growth, we in fact injure them, sometimes fatally.

In spite of his critique, Levinas seeks a safe space inside western thought that offers hospitality to the "Other." Ultimately, he fails, though there is much we may learn from him that allows us to create safer schools and classrooms for dangerous discourse. Levinas thinks it is possible to establish relations with the "Other" while respecting its alterity (see p. 42). He believes conversation provides a safe distance and medium of contact between the same and the "Other" (see p. 39). Levinas argues genuine conversation is unconstrained by thought or "the unfolding of a prefabricated internal logic" associated with regimes of truth and reason (p. 73). Levinas does not think it possible to entirely liberate dialogue from the constraining *logos* that it may yield "pure" knowledge, though it may yield astonishment, new knowledge, new experience, and growth. Supposedly, it is only theory as "the logos of being" that is such that the Other's alterity with regard to the knower vanishes (p. 42). The latter kind of theoretical knowing leads Levinas to deny the primacy of the knowing relation in favor of ethics.

Levinas asserts the primacy of ethical relations over knowing or ontological relations. For him, "The relation between the same and the other is not always reducible to knowledge of the other by the same" (p. 28). Instead, our primary relation is ethical: The strangeness of the "Other," his irreducibility to my thoughts and my possessions, is accomplished "as a calling into question of my spontaneity, as ethics" (p. 43). We desire the "Other" in their transcendence, but that does not mean we ontologically need them or even love them in any romantic sense. It involves hospitality or welcoming the other, though it has possibilities beyond that, not all of which we should welcome. Because for Levinas, our best relation with the "Other" is one of desire, our primary relation to "Others" is actually ethical-erotic. There is a profound precedence for this in the history of western thought. Levinas identifies the most influential when he indicates that it is here we encounter the Platonic idea of "the Good" that lies beyond "Being" (p. 293). The primacy of ethics over epistemological or even ontological relations is profoundly entrenched in western culture, though largely ignored by philosophers.

Levinas champions dialogue as the way to achieve transcendence before the face of the Other:

> It is therefore to receive from the Other beyond the capacity of the I, which means exactly; to have the idea of infinity. The relation with the Other, or Conversation, is . . . an ethical relation; but inasmuch as it is welcomed this conversation is a teaching. (p. 51)

Levinas thinks he can locate within the *logos* and metaphysics of western philosophy a healthy, analgesic conversation in a place apart from painful, potentially fatal dialogues, much as some teachers think they can assure a safe place for dialogue in their classrooms. However, there are no such safe sites, though teachers should strive to create safer spaces. Teachers should approach teacher-student dialogues with the assumption that students have a great deal to teach as well as learn. Good teaching is always transactional, which is not to say both parties learn the same thing. In the case of teaching the "Other," such reciprocity in teaching is especially important.

Surprisingly, our relation to the "Other" is not transactional for Levinas; it is hierarchical: "To recognize the Other is to give . . . to the master, to the lord . . . in a dimension of height" (75). The structure Levinas describes here is that of Master and Slave described in Hegel's (1807/1977) *Phenomenology of Spirit*, Section, IV a. According to Hegel, only the slave grows in such relations. Master/slave relations are sadly relevant to education because they permeate the educational hierarchy from student, to teacher, to principal, to superintendent, to politicians. In the discourse of education, technocratic masters merely repeat a calculative version of the rational discourse of modernity, e.g., accountability that reduces individual student differences to the same ciphers, norms, and standards that satisfy the purposes of the "free" market. The teachers who do not burn out, or students who do not drop out, grow in knowledge, if not in power. The slaves of technocratic discourse (students, staff, and teachers) often know the master far better than he knows himself. The fact that the social construction of the caring professions (teaching, nursing, and counseling) is that of silence and self-sacrifice, if not self-annihilation, only compounds the problem.

Often, the silent are active participants in the discourse. Ironically, these silent participants are often the only ones actually participating in a dialogue, so they are the only ones actually learning. Eventually, though, when they hear the same things constantly repeated it stops being a dialogue for them too. That is why many minority students become pedagogy-resistant, seek out their own affinity groups for dialogue, or become silenced nonparticipants.

Values and ideals of right action often express themselves ontologically as norms, standards, and hierarchies. Likewise, care and sympathy often disguise ontological violence. Teachers may humiliate by the glance of supervision, discipline, and control disguised as self-transcendent acts of care, kindness, and sympathy.

While I do not agree with Levinas that we can totally eliminate violence, it is still possible to approach the "Other" in a less violent "metaphysical" manner, to use Levinas's language, that offers respect, wonder, and the possibility of creating meaning and understanding with the "Other," thereby, satisfying the human eros for growth. Approaching the "Other" as if a dialogue can occur enhances the possibility it will. Similarly, it is a condition of knowledge and understanding, including self-knowledge, that we test its vulnerably before the tribunal of the "Other" and other situations. All claims are contingent and falsifiable. Further, I believe we know ourselves only insofar as we know the "Other" and the "Other" only insofar as we know ourselves. We may add such imperatives as these to the idea of the human eros because they call forth growth through expanded relationship. Such an approach requires risk, openness, and vulnerability; the dangers for all are greatest in such circumstance, though the possibilities for creative growth are also at their greatest.

Derrida's Deconstruction of Levinas

Derrida acknowledges he "was fascinated and attracted by the intellectual journey of Levinas," especially his "posing the question of the other" (quoted in Kearney, 1984, pp. 107–108). We may even read his deconstruction of Levinas (1978a) in *Violence and Metaphysics: An Essay on the Thought of Emmanuel Levinas* as homage to a mentor. Levinas thinks he can entirely separate violent forms of philosophical discourse (*logos*), ontology, and theory from nonviolent forms. He also constructs the "Other" as absolute alterity incommensurable with the concept of the self-same (ipseity). For Derrida, all these dualisms do is varnish over the violence, thereby making matters worse. In contrast, Derrida's deconstruction seeks to expose the violence hidden in all of western philosophy, thereby troubling speech while speaking beyond the silence.

Clearly, Derrida also wants to affirm some notion of the radical "Other" while defending them from violence as much as possible. He does so by deconstructing the logocentrism, phallocentrism, and phonocentrism along with the idea of fixed and unalterable centers of power that control all discourse. Derrida (1978b) also deconstructs the metaphysics of presence, but he does not dispose of it because he thinks such a total discontinuity with our past is impossible:

> There is no sense in doing without the concepts of metaphysics in order to shake metaphysics. We have no language—no syntax and no lexicon—which is foreign to this history; we can pronounce not a single destructive proposition which has not already had to slip into the form, the logic, and the implicit postulations of precisely what it seeks to contest. (pp. 280–281)

I detect a passionate ambivalence in Derrida; he recognizes we must live with the tensions of our linguistic inheritance because culture has us before we have it. That means that almost any discourse will show the influence of western metaphysics and its tendency to obliterate difference. This is especially the case with respect to the hyper-rational discourses of the technocracies that control public schooling. Derrida, however, does try to find a working vocabulary beyond the usual philosophical structures and terms in hopes of compassionately ameliorating the eliminable violence.

Derrida champions an ambivalent, paradoxical, and inclusive both/and strategy to alleviate the violent exclusion of the "Other" in philosophical constructions. He does not want to deny the self-identity of concepts, only the claim they are impermeable barriers marking off the conceptual purity of X from everything that is not-X. As one commentator states:

> It is not that identity is drowned in otherness, but that it is *necessarily* open to it, contaminated by it. Yet the necessity or essential character of this contamination cannot

be named unless we first grasp the concept of essence or form [*eidos*] as purity, as pure positive self-identity. (Staten, 1984, p. 18)

This discerning commentary is especially relevant since Derrida (1978a) indicates, "according to Levinas, all violence is a violence of the concept" (p. 140). Derrida's Both/And strategy recognizes that purity (e.g., racial purity, Puritanism, and so forth) is oppressive, violent, and often cruel. We will discover Derrida's ambivalent both/and strategy at work repeatedly in his deconstruction of Levinas. Derrida realizes in a dangerous world we "both" need working concepts, including those derived from the *logos* of western philosophy, "and" that such concepts are themselves dangerous for those who use them. This stance closely resembles the position I advocate of passionate ambivalence and the pursuit of compassionate amelioration.

For Levinas, according to Derrida, "The face is presence, *ousia*" (p. 101). For Derrida, though, there is no realization of some substance, some transcendental signified outside the mediated play of language; that means there is no "pure unmediated . . . perfect self-presence" (p. 115). There are only linguistic mediation, speech, and signs. There is no immediate possession of meaning, knowledge, or anything else and there is no immediate recognition of the face of the absolutely infinite otherness. Similarly, the "Other" is never entirely incommensurable. However complete, fixed, or finished one thinks their system may be there are always other possibilities, other interpretations, which is one of the things successful dialogues across difference may disclose even in the absence of understanding.

Derrida does not think we can eliminate violence in dialogue. Justifying this stance requires plumbing the depths of the very possibility of discourse and thought, so I can only provide its bare outline here. Having taken the linguistic turn, Derrida finds there is no thought without language, which means the violence of philosophy (e.g., metaphysics and the *logos*) infects all western thought. We cannot, contra Levinas, somehow find an absolutely safe space within philosophy, or simply leap out of our culture so influenced by it. Any child that does not engage in discourse will not come to have a mind or a self and therefore, ironically, will never think, know, or suffer the violence of the *logos*. Unfortunately, they will also never know the joy of being a *Homo sapiens* in its etymological sense of *sapientia*. Although education is the violence of the *logos*, I would still rather eat of the tree of knowledge, even if it means banishment of my mate and me from some nonlinguistic Eden.

Derrida rejects the binary structure of the *logos* along with its formal laws (e.g., the propositions: "A and not A" is always false, "A or not A" is always true). Without the pure, unmediated, and certain presence of self-identity, such immutable laws of correct Reason cannot function. For Derrida (1964/1978a), there is no simple absolute inside or outside to the "philosophical logos" (p. 112). That means, contra Levinas, "the infinite . . . cannot be stated," and we must acknowledge "the original finitude of speech and of whatever befalls it" (p. 113). We cannot use language, discourse, or thought, to capture something infinite exterior to it such as the absolutely infinite "Other." There are no transcendent places of frictionless face-to-face discourse. Similarly, there is no "Other" so transcendent that we may exercise no power over them, or they over us. Often, supposedly transcendent ideals conceal the practice of violence by placing actions in supernal realm beyond space, time, and circumstance (for example, actual classrooms and communities). Power over, power to, and power with always remain in place for better as well as worse. Derrida asserts, "As soon as one attempts to think Infinity as a positive plenitude . . . the other becomes unthinkable, impossible, unutterable" (p. 115). This does not mean we cannot recognize alterity, only that it is never beyond language or thought. We have no positive conception of any such thing as the infinite "Other": All we can do is think about the "in-finite," which is the negation of the finite things we can think.

Derrida asserts that the "distinction between discourse and violence always will be an inaccessible horizon. Nonviolence would be the telos, and not the essence of discourse" (p. 117). The core of discourse is violence, its "telos is nondiscourse: peace as a certain silence, a certain beyond of speech, a certain possibility, a certain silent horizon of speech" (p. 117). This is a "form of presence," something we cannot obtain, though we may properly pursue peace as an ideal through discourse, as Derrida does. Silence forced upon students by a totalized discourse establishes the kind of peace the authors featured in the present volume find disturbing because it conceals violence. Jones (this volume) shows that many prize silence because it provides peaceful respite from the relentless demands they disclose themselves through active participation in the classroom *logos*. Such "dialogues" are just disguised soliloquies because they ultimately reduce otherness and difference to the sameness of their sanctioned norms, categories, and identities. Meanwhile, Li (this volume) shows that silence is simply a moment in a continuous conversation. Ironically, there is an important sense in which silence is not a moment in the *logos*, but rather its "Other." For instance, silence often signals ignorance (i.e., the inability to participate in a dialogue), pausing to think before entering a dialogue is valued more than listening, and the only reason to listen is so you may speak better.

Derrida believes, "language can only tend toward justice by acknowledging and practicing the violence within it" (p. 117). Paradoxically, acting on such acknowledgement involves "Violence against violence" (p. 117). Teachers who seek to ameliorate violence take this approach instead of attempting the impossible task of guaranteeing a safe space. The question is always, "is the violence we take against violence in fact less violent than the violence we would allay." Does it actually ameliorate the situation? Levinas's ideal of the ethical good beyond knowledge (what

Derrida identifies as the classical Greek *epekeina tes ousias;* i.e., the substance of justice) is a valuable guide, but because the violence of the *logos* also infects this concept of the Good, Derrida finds it, too, is violent, though tending toward amelioration. In any discourse, it is wise to wonder whose ideal of the good controls the conversation. Levinas clearly recognizes the inevitability of conflict but thinks he can completely pacify it with the *logos* of Conversation.

Notice that Derrida's stance on discourse, sameness, and absolute, infinite alterity depends on the inclusive both/and characteristic of deconstruction. We find the same both/and working below as Derrida continues his deconstruction of Levinas's construction of the "Other." Derrida begins by noting, "to make the other an alter ego, Levinas says frequently, is to neutralize its absolute alterity" (p. 123). He does not think there is any such infinite otherness; therefore, he concludes:

> The other as alter ego signifies the other as other, irreducible to *my* ego, precisely because it is an ego [has an intentional structure], because it has the form of ego. The egoity of the other permits him to say "ego" as I do; and this is why he is Other. . . . Dissymmetry itself would be impossible without this symmetry. (p. 125)

Complete incommensurability implies complete unknowability, unrecognizability, and unrealizability, which would mean the "Other" does not appear to challenge, call out, or resist us.

Linguistic violence is the price we pay to have a mind. If there is a site or nonsite beyond the bounds of western philosophy where we may have a mind and a self nonviolently, we in the West will not arrive until we escape our history. Ignoring history is merely invisible violence. Perhaps nonviolence is the telos, though not the essence, of discourse; if so, Derrida contends, "eschato*logy* is not possible, except *through violence*. This infinite passage through violence is what is called history" (p. 130). He agrees with Levinas (1961/1995) that there are "ruptures of history" and that when "man truly approaches the Other he is uprooted from history" (p. 52). When our students and we approach each other in respect and wonder in our discourses, the consequences may displace us all from personal as well as cultural history, with unpredictable consequences. About all we may be sure of is many truths and values are doomed; any original thought places some part of an apparently stable world in peril and no one can guarantee what will emerge in its place. In spite of our best efforts, Derrida does not think anyone can fully escape the history of philosophy, though we may disturb ourselves by discourse with the "Other". Unfortunately, due to our own enculturation, we will bring our violence with us to every dialogue, or remain forever silent, but then there is no assurance the "Other" will not bring their violence with them.

Passionately Ambivalent Reflections on Liberalism, the Logos, *and Classroom Discourse*[4]

The *logos* (as speech) underwrites the First Amendment of the U.S. Constitution, which guarantees every individual the "right" of free speech. In recent years, this principle has become the safeguard for the "right" to engage in hateful and abusive speech largely directed toward people and principles that appear different from those of the cultural elites that founded the nation. While it authorizes many to speak, it also destroys any genuine possibility of free and open discourse for many others. Hate speech is devastating in the classroom. Still, the First Amendment is a form of violence against the yet worse violence of laws written against the possibility of any nonconforming speech. We should not forget that while many experience it as a colonizing speech code, people who suffered colonial rule wrote it. The best attitude toward it is one of passionate ambivalence that strives to compassionately ameliorate the code's residual violence through constitutional reconstruction.[5] Simplistic either/or thinking could lead us to reject the principle entirely, which would prove disastrous.

Many liberal thinkers such as John Stuart Mill (1859/1975) seek to go beyond merely the right to speak:

> In the case of any person whose [rational] judgment is really deserving of confidence, how has it become so? Because he has kept his mind open to criticism on his opinions and conduct. Because it has been his practice to listen to all that could be said against him. . . . He has felt, that the only way in which a human being can make some approach to knowing the whole of a subject, is by hearing what can be said about it by persons of every variety of opinion, and studying all modes in which it can be looked at by every character of mind. (p. 21)

I endorse the emphasis on open-mindedness and listening as an antidote to violence, though they too can conceal violence. We may trace Mill's model to the Greek *agon* (meaning, literally, "a contest") where ideas confront each other in the market place of ideas. Plato's Socratic dialogues are antagonistic in precisely this sense. For those who do not build their cultural discourse games on confrontation, the very structure of such dialogues is offensive. The model assumes that doubting the "Other" and confronting their claims leads to truth and wisdom. For those whose conversational style presumes trying to believe what others say is valid for them, and possibly valid for us, or seeking to avoid confrontation, the dominant western approach to critical thinking offends or is impossible to use.[6] Furthermore, because the market place is not a neutral site of mediation, the contest is never fair.

Mill (1859/1975) goes on to state his ideal of listening when he suggests, "Not the violent conflict between parts of truth, but the quiet suppression of half of it, is the formidable evil; there is always hope when people are forced to listen to both sides; it is when they attend only to one that errors harden into prejudices" (p. 50). Following the *logos* leads Mill to presume there is only one true telling. Further, what does "forced to listen" mean, and who has the power to assure compliance? In violent conflict, it is the least powerful who suffer domination and silence. Alison Jones (this volume) exposes another kind of violence working in the opposite direction. By listening attentively to the "Other" in supposedly safe spaces, the privileged and powerful gain access to, knowledge about, and, hence, power over, the already exploited. She is right to observe that dialogue as a supposedly innocent and neutral mediator may readily lead to colonial surveillance and oppression. Michel Foucault's (1972/1980) idea of "power/knowledge" provides a detailed analysis of how discourses can contribute to the construction of matrices of manipulation and domination. Frequently, confessional self-disclosure occurs in a putatively safe space, such as a classroom, which, in actuality, is often one of the primary sites of power, command, and control. To teach well teachers must know their students well, but while enlightening knowledge is power, power for and power with readily yield to the violence of power over. It is here that compassionate perception and moral imagination may matter most, but there is also pitiless perception and immoral imagination.

Open-mindedness and listening could leave the oppressed vulnerable to abuse while leaving the powerful with privileged information. There is a profound ambivalence here, because only open-mindedness and listening can satisfy the human eros. Mutual compassion, risk, and vulnerability (as well as a sense of humor) oriented toward the amelioration of a shared situation would go a long way toward the continuous reconstruction of communicative pluralistic democracy, but there is no absolute escape from the danger and violence in discourse.

Notes

1. Also see Garrison (1986).
2. See Siegel (1997).
3. Levinas is interested in the unique, individual personal ipsiety of the "Other" *("l'autrui")* not the "other" *("autre")* of things, ideas, etc. This sense of "the Other" is the primary subject of my paper. In the remainder of this essay, I will us the "Other" in quotes to indicate *l'autrui*.
4. This section expands on Garrison (1996).
5. A profound ambivalence already exists between the First and Fourteenth Amendments that could provide a lever for reconstruction.
6. Phelan and Garrison (1994) locate a gender bias in traditional "critical thinking" that privileges the "doubting game" over the "believing game" when both are necessary to understand and critique the position of another.

References

Alexander, T. (1993). The human eros. In J. Stuhr (ed). *Philosophy and the reconstruction of culture* (pp. 203–222). Albany: State University of New York Press.

Boler, M. (This volume). All speech is not free: The ethics of affirmative action pedagogy.

Derrida, J. (1978a). Violence and metaphysics: An essay on the thought of Emmanuel Levinas. In *Writing and difference* (pp. 79–153) (Alan Bass, Trans.). Chicago: The University of Chicago Press.

Derrida, J. (1978b). Structure, Sign, and Play in the Discourse of the Human Sciences. In *Writing and Difference* (pp. 278–293) (Alan Bass, Trans.). Chicago: The University of Chicago Press.

Foucault, M. (1980). *Power/knowledge.* New York: Pantheon Books. (Original work published in 1972)

Garrison, J. (1986). The paradox of indoctrination: A solution. *Synthese, 68,* 261–273.

Garrison, J. (1996). A Deweyan theory of democratic listening. *Educational Theory,* 429–451.

Hegel, G. W. F. (1977). *Phenomenology of sprit.* Oxford: Oxford University Press. (Original work published in 1807)

Jones, A. (This volume). Talking cure: The desire for dialogue.

Kearney, R. (Ed.). (1984). Deconstruction and the other. In *Dialogues with contemporary continental thinkers.* Manchester: Manchester University Press.

Levinas, E. (1995). *Totality and infinity.* Pittsburgh: Duquesne University Press. (Original work published in 1961)

Li, H. L. (This volume). Silences silencing silences.

Macmillan, C. J. B. (1983). On certainty and indoctrination. *Synthese, 56,* 363–372.

Mill, J. (1975). *On liberty.* New York: W. W. Norton and Company. (Original work published in 1859)

Phelan, A., J. Garrison (1994). Toward a gender-sensitive ideal of critical thinking. In Kerry S. Walters (Ed.) *Re-thinking reason: New perspectives in critical thinking* (pp. 81–97). Albany: New York State University Press.

Siegel, H. (1997). *Rationality redeemed? Further dialogues on an educational ideal.* New York: Routledge.

Staten, H. (1984). *Wittgenstein and Derrida.* Lincoln: University of Nebraska Press.

Wittgenstein, L. (1972). *On certainty.* New York: Harper & Row.

Barbara Houston

Democratic Dialogue: Who Takes Responsibility?

In this chapter I address the question of open and honest dialogue among students of difference about large-scale problems of social injustice, with an eye to how we might assist students, and ourselves, in taking responsibility for such problems. By their nature, these are pervasive social problems of which it is true to say that no one of us caused them. They are also problems that will stay entrenched and likely worsen if we do not do something about them.[1]

The difficulties in fostering open and honest dialogue across significant differences among students in educational settings, especially dialogue about social injustice, have led to serious questions about its feasibility. For example, other authors in this volume offer reasons for thinking that, in our present circumstances, democratic dialogue is deeply ambiguous and morally suspect (deCastell, this volume; Jones, this volume).

In fact, there are numerous reasons why democratic dialogue among students has become suspect:

- It is not easy to gain any sort of shared understanding among the participants of what the project entails and who might benefit;
- Those who are least able to control the shape, direction, and determination of the "success" of such dialogue may not only be unenthusiastic about it, they may also be, rightly, suspicious of it;
- With candid speech about matters of social injustice there is the possibility of increasing harm inasmuch as it can deepen the dilemma of repression and abuse of subjugated groups (Matsuda et al., 1993); and

- Given the momentous institutional pressures against it, the political and educational skill required, as well as the emotional difficulty associated with it, there may be few educators with the capacity to effectively cultivate democratic dialogue (Houston, 1994).

Nevertheless, there remain good reasons for attempting democratic dialogue. Perhaps the central reason is that it is hard to imagine how one might sustain democracy in its absence. Heesoon Bai (2001) addresses this issue by introducing the concept of intersubjectivity. She describes intersubjectivity as engaging "in the mutual sharing of thoughts, perceptions, values across individual differences" (p. 311); and she claims it is a characteristic required of people who aspire to democracy, i.e., to mutual governance. Bai reminds us of the fact that it is when people "interact with each other in *mutual inquiry, consultation, and deliberation* with the aim of arriving at a *common good* that we have democracy" (p. 308, original emphasis). Indeed, as she notes, the power of democracy lies in the wisdom that emerges from putting our minds and hearts together. It is not that we need to aim for or achieve unity of thought; we expect conflict. What matters is to have forums for exploring conflicts, ways of engaging with one another about the conflicts, which do not systematically disadvantage some participants. This is the ideal; it is debatable how much we struggle to enact it, or how much we care to know when we are failing to attain it.

Central to democracy's enactment is a will to the common good, or "good will," and while there may be disagreement about exactly how we cultivate good will sufficient for democratic citizenship, it is recognized that there is a kind of relatedness integral to it. Bai (2001) describes it this way:

Sharing our thoughts, perceptions, hopes, fears, desires, as well as the actual sweat of human labour is what makes us feel bonded to each other and makes us committed to promoting each other's well-being. Thus the meaning of, or the reasons for, mutual inquiry, consultation, and deliberation is that we share ourselves in words and in deeds. Dialogue wherein we share our minds and hearts, therefore, is the most fundamental activity of democracy. (p. 310)

My approach to the question of the value of democratic dialogue is built on the following premises. First, I agree with Bai that it is a "fundamental activity of democracy." Second, I believe we cannot compel moral goodness; we can only nurture it. In this regard, adopting a certain generosity toward human frailty and mistakes is a more likely route to success. If we cannot be open about our mistakes, it is unlikely that we will have much opportunity to correct them. Third, education is an arena where, nominally at least, we learn what our mistakes might be and how to correct them. If we discourage dialogue about these matters in schools, education risks losing even the possibility of transformative value, for everyone. Thus, I support attempting democratic dialogue about matters of social injustice in education, making sure that the challenge of it and the obstacles to it become part of the discussion.

In order to address some of the obstacles, I propose we look more closely at the implicit assumptions about responsibility, which plague most efforts to engage students in democratic dialogue about matters of social justice. These assumptions underlie two of the most common debilitating obstacles:

- an entrenched public resistance on the part of students to taking on such problems, and
- a kind of moral paralysis when they do attempt to take them on.

For example, in her BBC Reith lectures, Patricia Williams (1997) cites both of these obstacles to dialogue across differences of race.

[T]he eradication of prejudice, the reconciling of tensions across racial, ethnic, cultural and religious lines depends [in part]. . .upon eradicating the troublesome attitudinal divide between the paralyzing anxiety of well-meaning "white guilt" and the smoldering unhappiness of blacks who dare not speak their mind. (p. 61)

As Williams indicates, resistance to discussing these issues and a sense of being stymied around them arise among the dominant and privileged, as well as the subordinate and marginalized. Depending upon which particular form of social injustice happens to be at the center of our attention, we can find ourselves shifting from one of these groups to another. Thus, while my arguments for the adoption of certain strategies with respect to responsibility are designed to encourage members of dominant or privileged groups to take more social responsibility, I also see my recommendations as having wider applicability. They have wider applicability, I believe, because we all have responsibilities to take up in response to social injustices, however they may differ. With respect to any such responsibilities, the tacit assumptions clustered around them, and the blameworthiness that attaches to us in virtue of them, can be debilitating. Among the many large-scale problems of social injustice, I shall focus in this chapter on only one, that of race.

It is no secret that there is widespread resistance to taking on responsibility for problems of racial injustice. Sandra Bartky (2002), speaking in the context of the United States, and of white people, asks: "What goes on in the minds of "nice" white people which allows them to ignore the terrible effects of racism, and to the extent that these effects are recognized at all, to deny that they bear any responsibility for their perpetration" (p. 151).

Wholly cognizant of her own role in perpetuating social injustice, Bartky describes what she calls "phenomenologies of denial" (p. 154) and sets forth a typology of the people who employ them. Among them she includes the fantasists who believe that racism is already overcome; the clueless "[who] have no effective understanding of racism at all" (p. 156); the self-deceivers, who do know a great deal about racism and who, according to Bartky, are culpable but not ignorant because they deny "that they bear any responsibility either for maintaining or for perpetuating the racial caste hierarchy" (p. 159); and the fearful. As Bartky acknowledges, it would be a mistake to underestimate how much fear can be operative in our "not knowing what one knows" (p. 163). We may fear that if we fully open ourselves to the misery of others, we will be swallowed up by it, tossed into an "emotional abyss so vast that it would paralyze our ability to act (p. 163).[2]

This typology captures some of the phenomenologies of denial that arise in classrooms when we undertake dialogue about race issues. While Bartky focuses on our unwillingness to acknowledge our complicity in perpetuating human misery, I want to start one step further back with an assumption logically prior to hers. My assumption is that most of us do not want to perpetuate human misery, and so, in that sense, I assume to be speaking here of "decent people."[3] I start here, within the territory of moral psychology, and ask: Where might we look for personal obstacles to bearing responsibility? What hinders us at this level?

I propose it is the very concept of responsibility employed to hold us accountable that hinders us. My central thesis is that the prevalent public resistance and moral paralysis may be explained, in large part, by what I call our default notion of moral responsibility. My main recommendation will be that if we are to engage students in dialogue across difference about problems of social injustice, and if in such dialogues we want to maintain or cultivate a sense of agency in addressing these problems, then we need to become more adept at shifting perspectives on taking responsibility.

What I am calling the "default notion," Marion Smiley (1992) calls "the modern concept of moral responsibility."[4] Relying upon Smiley's argumentation, I want to direct attention to certain features of this inherited notion of moral responsibility, some apparent, some tacit, which underlie the moral emotional difficulties I am investigating. Perhaps the most important feature of our notion of moral responsibility is the way in which we keep it distanced from conventional norms and practices. If we are to see morality as an independent source for critique of conventions including legal ones, then moral responsibility must be seen as beyond, outside, not wholly encompassed by any social community's conventions, including conventional blaming practices. Joel Feinberg (1970) reminds us that the terminology of *moral* obligation, *moral* guilt and *moral* responsibility expresses a "conception of a 'real' theoretical possibility distinct from a practical responsibility 'relative' to the purposes and values of a particular legal system . . ." Thus, moral responsibility, he says, is a matter of "judgements which are in no way forced by practical considerations," and they impute "an absolute responsibility within the power of the agent" (p. 30).

Judgments of moral responsibility then, inasmuch as they impute the possibility of action within the power of the agent, can resemble judgments of fact. However, their implications are much broader than any empirical claim because these attributions of moral responsibility carry within them "a moral judgement about the individual in question: that she is morally blameworthy for having brought about harm" (Smiley, 1992, p. 74). William Frankena (1963) elucidates this fusion of causation and accusation, characteristic of the modern concept of responsibility:

> Saying that X was responsible for Y seems, at first, to be a causal, not a moral, judgement; and one might, therefore, be inclined to say that "X was responsible for Y" simply means "x caused y," perhaps with the qualification that he did so voluntarily, intentionally, etc. But to say that X is responsible for Y is not merely to make a causal statement of a special kind. . . . It is to say that it would be right to blame or otherwise punish him." (p. 56)

According to Smiley, this conflation of causation and moral blameworthiness is the "distinguishing mark" (p. 75) of the modern concept of moral responsibility. The operating assumption is this: Given the absence of excusing conditions, which undermine the judgment of causation, a person who is responsible is *ipso facto* blameworthy. The implications of such a view are serious, though not always fully acknowledged: The individual's agency becomes the source of moral blameworthiness. Further, "since it is a judgement of the individual's moral worth, it cannot refer simply to her actions but must refer to her as a person" (Smiley, 1992, p. 75). Jonathan Glover (1970) clearly articulates this view that moral blameworthiness constitutes a moral fact about the worth of persons as moral agents. He states unequivocally, to say that someone is morally blameworthy for some state of affairs "is to say that he is a bad person" (p. 96).

We can see how attributions of moral responsibility as thus characterized entail something of a slippery slope where we slide almost imperceptibly from judgments about causation to assessments of the worth of persons. Specifically, we can note the following separable features:

- judgments of moral responsibility are removed from and assumed to be independent of conventional social and legal norms;
- judgments of causation are fused with moral praise/blame; which means
- moral blameworthiness becomes a function (solely) of individual agency which carries with it
- a judgment of the (intrinsic) worth of the person.

These features of the modern concept of responsibility are based on stringent requirements for the assignment of moral responsibility: The individual will must be free, "wholly free of external determination" if it is to be the source of blameworthiness; and the will must be capable of being intrinsically good or bad (Smiley, 1992, p. 78). Given these requirements, this default concept of moral responsibility is not one that we can coherently employ in the social political arena which abounds with tenuous causal connections between individuals and social harm to groups. Who could reasonably claim that problems that fall under the term *racism* are reducible to individual agency? Who nowadays could or would defend the claim that our wills, if it makes sense to talk about individual wills, can be intrinsically good or bad? Nevertheless, we do apply this notion of responsibility, or, more accurately, misapply it, all the time. Not without consequences, however.

There are significant consequences for our moral emotional lives when we make such attributions of moral responsibility without being able to meet the assumed requirements the modern notion relies upon. There are, as it were, psychological side effects to this conceptual incoherence and its misapplication. Two of these side effects are the problems under discussion, namely those of social resistance and moral paralysis. We can get a sense of how these psychological side effects operate if we look at Sandra Bartky's discussion of "guilt by privilege," a not uncommon "charge" students or instructors make.

Bartky describes "guilt by privilege" as a variant of "guilt by complicity" where one is complicitous with the existing structure of the established social-political order. However confused or opaque the referent for social-political order may be, the key idea is that "I am guilty by virtue of my relationship to wrong doing, a relationship that I did not create but which I have not severed either" (p. 142). Bartky claims, "the very structure of everyday life places the relatively privileged in a morally compromised position, whether we know we are in it or not. One can be guilty without feeling guilty and without having authored the social arrangements that involve one in complicity" (p. 146). She says of herself, "On my view I am guilty simply by virtue of being who and what I am: a white woman, born into an aspiring middle-class family in a racist and class-ridden society" (p. 146). This entire line of thinking, and blaming, exemplifies the modern concept of responsibility at work, specifically in its suggestion that blameworthiness is simply a matter of fact: "There is complicity involved. . . . My role in the maintenance of an unjust social order is a fact, *whether I recognize it or not*" (p. 142, original emphasis).

Understandably, because they do not want to feel they are guilty of perpetuating human misery, Bartky's students are not receptive to such judgments. She notes:

This is undoubtedly the reason that my white middle-class students respond regularly with anger, defensiveness, or denial when I suggest to them that we whites enjoy privileges that are systematically denied to non-whites. [They say] "I've never abused or insulted a black person!" or "My parents came here thirty years ago from Croatia: my forebears were peasants not slaveholders. (p. 141)

Bartky acknowledges that "My students are onto something, namely the distinction between having done something wrong and having done nothing wrong"(p. 142). Even so, she insists on making what she calls the counterintuitive claim that "one can be guilty *without having done anything wrong*"(p. 142, original emphasis).[5]

Another feature of the modern concept of responsibility emerges here. The guilt Bartky assigns is quite like intrinsic guilt inasmuch as the efforts or agency of the individual can never expunge it. Bartky asks: "How much effort on the part of a person will cancel her complicity, hence remove her guilt? How can this cancellation ever be complete?" (p. 147) Her answer, with respect to "guilt by privilege," is clear; "in many respects it cannot be cancelled" (p. 148). She says, "There are some inequalities from which we cannot entirely divorce ourselves no matter how hard we try. White skin privilege is a case in point. . . . one cannot have clean hands where the polity is unclean" (p. 148).

It is not surprising then that students feel they need to resist this notion if they are not to be defeated by it. What Bartky appears to miss in her diagnosis of students' responses is the import of this responsibility judgment for their sense of worth as persons. They reject the implication that they are bad persons because of their relation to a social order over which they lack control. It is this implied judgment of their worth as persons, I believe, that is one primary source of her students' resistance. We can sense the likelihood of this if we try on an alternative assessment of responsibility. What if, for example, we were to say to our students: "You are involved in something wrong and you are not being judged"? This alternative assessment seems less likely to invoke resistance and more likely to elicit curiosity, perhaps even some desire to meet the challenge of conceiving and enacting an alternative.[6]

Consideration of this alternative assessment, "You are involved in something wrong and you are not being judged," can highlight the ways in which the modern default concept of responsibility eclipses key assumptions and implicit norms that are needed to make judgments of blameworthiness coherent. In the modern concept these are smuggled into the so-called "factual" judgments. Bartky's claim, "My role in the maintenance of an unjust social order is a fact, whether I recognize it or not," seems to establish blameworthiness. However, even if we grant the judgment about an unjust social order, we still can ask: What is it that makes me blameworthy here?

A number of questions would need to be asked and answered. For instance, where do we decide to begin and end the causal chain we think is relevant? Is my role in maintaining an unjust order a function of my agency? If "one cannot have clean hands where the polity is unclean," who and what determine the relevant polity? Does everyone in the polity have dirty hands, including the oppressed? If intrinsic guilt attaches to a person by virtue of their being irrevocably attached or identified with a particular community, how do we determine the community with which they ought to be identified? What defines the boundaries of this community within which I am privileged? If my parents came here from Croatia, does that mean I bear the same responsibility as those whose great-grandparents were slaveholders? Answers to questions such as these seem to be required as a support for coherent blame. The point to notice is that they invoke norms. However, in our current default concept these questions and their implicit norms have been swallowed up by the so-called "fact" of "my role in the maintenance of an unjust social order."

Without an accepted or agreed upon framework within which to raise and consider these sorts of questions, judgments of blameworthiness, when they are not resisted, can be paralyzing. Consider the example of Marilyn Frye (1990) who describes herself as wholly demoralized by self-blame in her efforts to respond constructively to criticisms of herself and her work as racist.

> It all combined to precipitate me into profound and unnerving distrust of myself. All of my ways of knowing seemed to have failed me—my perception, my common sense, my good will, my anger, honor and affection, my intelligence and insight. Just as walking requires something fairly sturdy and firm underfoot, so being an actor in the world requires a foundation of ordinary moral and intellectual confidence. Without that, we don't know how to be or how to act; we become strangely stupid. . . . If you want to be good and you don't know good from bad, you can't move. (p. 133)

Frye's comments testify to the emotional fallout that can occur when the judgments of blame we incur from others and ourselves involve a misapplication of the modern concept of moral responsibility. In cases of both resistance and paralysis, it is our worth as persons that feels threatened or defeated.

The question arises whether we can side-step this sort of resistance and sense of defeat in our dialogues if we take a different perspective on responsibility, a perspective that increases our sense of agency. Claudia Card (1996) notes two distinguishable perspectives associated with the phrase "taking responsibility:" first, the "backward looking" or evaluator's perspective, and second, the "forward looking" or agent's perspective (p. 26). The backward-looking perspective is the one we have seen at work in the Bartky and Frye examples. This perspective, common in contemporary Anglo-American philosophy is concerned primarily with attributions of blameworthiness, determining who bears responsibility in order to assign blame. It is said to be a backward-looking perspective because the focus is on looking back to some previous action in order to judge it. Conversely, the forward-looking perspective, "embodies a perspective of agency" (p. 26). It involves the taking on of responsibility, "which can be for what has not yet occurred or has not yet been done" (p. 25). Bernard Williams (1981) has called it "the view from here" (p. 33). Of central interest to us is the point that in the forward looking sense, when we take (on) responsibility for something, say problems of social injustice, there is no assumption that we produced these problems.

These two perspectives on taking responsibility are exemplified in the exchanges between a man's backward looking perspective and a woman's forward looking perspective in Adrienne Rich's poem "From an Old House in America" (1984). The man, having recently realized how he is implicated in social relations and structures harmful to women, asks such questions as "Will you punish me for history?," "Do you believe in collective guilt?" The woman gives the same reply to all of his questions, "What will you undertake?" (p. 220).

The woman reminds the man of his agency with the simple words, "what will you undertake." So too, rather than getting stuck in moral paralysis and social resistance to blame, rather than becoming fixated on our justifications for what we have or have not done, we can adopt a forward looking perspective on taking responsibility. We can acknowledge the problems and ask ourselves the question: what will I undertake?

Even when we adopt a forward-looking perspective on responsibility, however, and try to move beyond being stuck by judgments that we are bad persons because of what we do or do not do with respect to matters largely beyond our control, we often run into yet another psychological obstacle. This obstacle is the belief that taking on responsibility for problems of social injustice requires us to identify with the collectives within which we appear to be situated, especially when these collectives have harmed groups we aim to support.[7]

The pressure to so identify can come from those with whom we wish to offer solidarity, or from within ourselves. In any case, such pressure frequently meets with resistance and/or perplexity. Joel Feinberg (1968) gives voice to the perplexity when he comments on his inability to identify with other members of the white race. "I . . . am quite incapable of feeling . . . solidarity with all white men, a motley group of one billion persons who in my mind are no more an 'organization' than is the entire human race. I certainly feel no bonds to nineteenth century slave traders" (p. 677). Feinberg expresses both bewilderment and resistance; bewilderment about how one might identify as white, why one should, and resistance to identifying with a group of whom he morally disapproves. This echoes the similar protest from Bartky's student: "My parents came here thirty years ago from Croatia: my forebears are peasants not slaveholders."

For those of us who appear to belong to collectivities that have caused harm, does taking responsibility require us to identify with them? Some argue that we cannot avoid such identifications. They claim this need to identify becomes obvious when we consider the problems that arise if instead we try to take responsibility for problems of racism, sexism, or poverty by sympathetically identifying with the "victims," believing that through sympathetic identification we can better appreciate their hardships, sufferings, and humiliations and so are more likely to feel outrage and indignation on their behalf. This strategy of sympathetic identification, however, runs into difficulties. The "victims" reject the outrage on their behalf because they still see the sympathetic identifier as part of the group collectively responsible for the harm done to them. The argument in favor of identification with our privileged group(s) turns on the need to acknowledge how others see us so that we can begin to understand their moral claims against us. As Campbell (2002) argues, in so identifying, "We may at least take ourselves to be addressed by others in ways that might motivate seeing how we are understood by them" (p. 12).

The necessity of receptivity, the necessity of moral addressability by others is critical in democratic dialogue. Even so, does it require our identification with groups, especially those we experience as alien? Undoubtedly, in some cases, these forms of identification can aid us in the way Campbell suggests. However, it is not obvious that such identifications are *necessary* in order to make ourselves morally addressable or receptive. What is obvious, however, is that when people encounter pressure to claim what they experience as an alien or inappropriate identity, the same sorts of bewilderment, moral paralysis, and resistance show up that arose with the default concept of blameworthiness. If our concern is with moral agency, we again need to find a way to avoid getting stuck here.

At this point, I want to suggest we consider adopting a different strategy. I propose we see taking responsibility with respect to these problems as a matter of taking responsibility for oneself, not necessarily as a matter of identifying with any particular group. This would be to persist with the forward-looking perspective on taking responsibility, emphasizing the agent's perspective rather than the evaluator's. The worries about addressability or responsiveness, recognition of interdependence, and acknowledgment of historical continuities do not disappear; but we may herein find a constructive rather than a resistant strategy for working with them.

When I suggest that in democratic dialogue we might construe taking responsibility for social problems as a matter of taking responsibility for oneself, I want to find a way to focus on what it means to begin right here where we are, in the present, in the midst of all our current resistances, conflicts, confusions, and tensions. I see this as the place to start, the place where we can allow, and not forget, that we are more than our identifications, our own and those others attribute to us.

Taking responsibility for oneself, in this sense, involves acknowledging our situatedness and location, material, historical, and bodily specificity, the interconnections between our own well-being and the existence of others. Taking responsibility for ourselves recognizes that our existence cannot be severed from, or remains fungible with, the lives of others past and future. It is a matter primarily of recognizing and dealing with my own resistances, the internal conflicts, and tensions, which if unacknowledged can operate as obstacles to my being responsive to others. Thus, I believe, it can become a way for me to be more responsive to others.

Nevertheless, one cannot responsibly recommend such a strategy for dialogue about problems of social injustice without acknowledging three significant facts.

1. We are all both persons, individual moral agents with the ability to make choices, and members of different collectivities or "mobs" as Dwight Boyd (1998) calls them when he notes that: "However much I am, and experience myself to be a unique individual, I am in fact already part of a mob. . . . That is, I am unavoidably part of something that is doing something to me, for me, through me, as me" (p. 13).

2. Respectful relations across differences require all parties to acknowledge each other as both unique persons and members of groups.

3. It is typical of majority or privileged persons that they/we want to see themselves/ourselves as "human beings" or unique individuals, while minority or subordinated people want to see them/us as members of groups responsible for injustice. Furthermore, one of the privileges of the majority/dominant group is that we can determine when to invoke our identity as individuals and when to invoke or simply enjoy the benefits without noticing our identity as a group member. Minority or subordinate people do not have this choice about which aspect of their identity is salient; and frequently members of the majority or dominant group are the ones to make that determination. Still, if identification with the collectivity is something we want or even believe we need in our dialogues about how to effectively tackle problems of social injustice, we are unlikely to get it if we insist on it. Such insistence tends to increase resistance.

On the surface it might also sound as though I am recommending a strategy that could land us in a worse dead-end, a narcissistic fixation on one's own character rather than on the social harms that need to be corrected. I do not deny this can be a risk of my strategy. However, we also know the risks of persisting with the backward looking perspective. Being stuck in blame, self-blame, or blame from others, can also keep us fixed in the wrong way—focused on ourselves and our endless justifications for why we are not to blame.[8]

One virtue of the strategy I'm suggesting is that it may make it easier for people to examine their own hostilities and resistances if they do so as a matter of being accountable to themselves. This is part of a strategy that Claudia Card (1996) has advocated for those with diminished agency as a result of their personal history.[9] While it may seem odd to claim that we all suffer diminished moral agency, I think it is not so far off to think of everyone in this way when we are talking about major social problems, which leave most of us feeling powerless. With respect to such social problems as racism, we do all face a state of diminished agency.

Even so, someone might ask: What if an individual's sense of the self for which she is responsible is bounded, limited, separated; what if she does not see herself as needing to be responsive to others, in particular these others? Indeed as Megan Boler (1999) and Margaret Urban Walker (1998) have argued, it is likely that many of us will have just such a conditioned sense of self, where even our emotions have been politically shaped in part by the dominant subordinate structuring of our social relations. It seems to me that this is exactly the reason to start here, at home, with ourselves. This is where we begin the work of self-knowledge and self-understanding in connection with social problems of injustice. It is where structural analyses can get their grip. It is not, of course, the place to end our work. Kierkegaard (1987) and Nel Noddings (2002), among others, remind us constantly that the life impulse is in the subjectivity of persons, not in theories, obligations, and structures. What Kierkegaard calls "double reflection"[10] is a rethinking of the structures within which one finds oneself, reevaluating them in such a way that one's thinking leads to action. I am arguing that, with respect to problems of social injustice, an explicit shift to the notion of taking responsibility for oneself can provide us a way to assist our students, and ourselves, avoid inauthenticity and practice Kierkegaard's double reflection.

In the end, not everyone will be motivated to engage with problems of social injustice or to take on responsibility for these problems in the same way. The way we choose seems to me to be less important than whether or not we engage constructively with the problems. For those who get stuck around "identification," their sense of agency might depend upon their construing the taking of responsibility for social problems as a matter of taking responsibility for their own character. Not everyone will be engaged by this move, but for some this shift in their concept of taking responsibility could be crucial to their staying with the attempts to do something about seemingly intractable problems. Wendell Berry (1990) gives us a sense of how it might work. In noting that "History simply affords us too little evidence that anyone's individual protest is of any use" (p. 62), Berry adds: "Protest that endures, I think, is moved by a hope far more modest than that of public success; namely the hope of preserving qualities in one's own heart and spirit that would be destroyed by acquiescence" (p. 62).

Before concluding, I want to acknowledge and speak to two more obvious risks with my suggestions.[11] While my proposed shifts in responsibility seem helpful in freeing up energy that is stuck. We do need to ask whether actions motivated from these senses of taking responsibility are likely to change, or even address, the underlying structures of inequity and oppression because, obviously, one of the dangers in this terrain is that those of us in positions of privilege want to feel less bad, not guilty or maybe even virtuous. The risk is that we want to do this without losing the privileges that are part of the structure that is causing harm.

I believe some actions motivated by these senses of taking responsibility could contribute if only by prompting conversations and shifts in awareness that could lead to such change. They will do so, however, only if we can remain alert to the possibility that underneath our good intentions is unrecognized self-interest that may have led to the inertness or resistance in the first place.

Another, perhaps even greater risk associated with my strategy is whether the two alternative senses of taking responsibility I have laid out are missing a recognition of just how interdependent we, as members of privileged groups, are with members of subordinate groups with whom we are trapped in an oppressive dynamic beyond our own choosing. As members of a privileged majority we are used to being able to take effective action, either on our own or with members of our own groups. However, with instances of large-scale social problems, if we want to move beyond a sense of paralysis or resistance, to move outside the dynamics of guilt and blame, we need our counterparts to also take responsibility. Because when we look beyond the power dynamics, when we look at the possibility of creating a different future, we require a different kind of relationship with those others who invoke such uncomfortable feelings in us now.

The legacy of harm entails alienation from our understanding of ourselves as moral beings, and from each other. Taking responsibility for oneself can help us to overcome the sense of alienation from ourselves. The best possibility, the one I hope for, is that it might also free us to reach for a different relationship with the other.

In sum, the democratic dialogue I envision will not only bring different notions of responsibility into play, it will also acknowledge different conceptions of the self at work in our thinking about responsibility and agency. Discussions about problems of social injustice that both implicate us and feel beyond our influence, when combined with a backward looking notion of responsibility that focuses on blame and accusation, can easily give rise to a sense of demoralization that manifests itself in resistance, denial, and/or moral inertia. At the heart of this demoralization is a hard truth. In one sense, the self is socially constituted as a mob-like individual who needs to come to terms with the fact that each of us is "unavoidably part of something that is doing something to me, for me, through me, as me" (Boyd, 1998, p. 13). My focus in this essay has been on how we might preserve the individual's sense of their capacity for taking responsibility in the face of large-scale social problems. In doing so I have relied upon a non-mob-like picture of the self. It is a worry that the two pictures seem incompatible.[12]

In the end, how responsible we actually are depends upon our capacity to act responsibly in both word and deed. Perhaps what we need is another picture altogether, a less dualistic one that highlights our interconnectedness, our interbeing, one that we experientially know to be a truer picture. We might then feel less burdened by responsibilities and more able to engage them. In dialogues where we share our minds and hearts, where we do not feel ourselves to be taken as a means to some political end, we might more readily bear the pain of each other's truth. Could such a picture emerge as the fruit of engagement in democratic dialogue?

Notes

1. An earlier version of my approach to these same issues can be found in Houston (2003).

2. Bartky herself offers some astute structural analyses to explain these forms of denial, while still insisting that such explanations do not let us off the hook. There is no question of either the importance or the necessity of grasping the structural features of the situation. However, I want to turn our attention to additional obstacles.

3. The phrase "decent people" I adopt from Norman Care (2000) who speaks of the moralized pain decent people feel and how our moral emotional nature moves us to seek relief from it. I take the term to refer to "good people of all races and ages, good people of good will" (Williams, 1997, p. 61).

4. With Smiley, I think it fair to say that this notion of responsibility is held by a great percentage of the secular population as well as by large numbers of contemporary Anglo-American philosophers who write about moral responsibility. Further, in the absence of a consciously articulated alternative notion of moral responsibility such as, for example, a Strawsonian account or a utilitarian concept of responsibility like that offered by Richard Brandt, the modern concept is, I believe, the inherited default notion within the western tradition. For an account of moral responsibility that, unlike "the modern concept," explains moral responsibility in terms of social practices and what he calls "reactive attitudes" see P. F. Strawson (1974). For attempts to develop a utilitarian conception of responsibility that leaves behind notions of causation and free will and concentrates on the consequences of blame for society see J. J. C. Smart (1961) and Richard Brandt (1969).

5. One might ask whether it is not more appropriate to claim that Bartky is rejecting the modern concept of responsibility, rather than misapplying it, inasmuch as she appears to be rejecting altogether the first requirement of causation. Bartky's discussion is more ambiguous than I can detail here. Sometimes she suggests that we are guilty because we have not severed our connection with wrongdoing, or have done nothing about the *persistence* of prejudice, thus strongly implying that we have done something wrong through our inaction. Further, she nowhere indicates that she rejects the modern concept of responsibility, so I assume for her, too, it is the default notion.

6. This is not to deny that the privileges that go with a given social order make it tempting to those who enjoy them to resist any quests for alternative arrangements.

7. This point is discussed in Sue Campbell's paper, "Emotion, memory and political identification," presented to the Canadian Society for Women in Philosophy, The University of Guelph, Guelph, Ontario, Canada, September 2002. For obvious reasons, Campbell calls this requirement "resistant identification." A point worth remembering is that the pressure to identify with the collectivities to which we belong is resisted by members of subordinate and marginalized as well as dominant and privileged groups. All subsequent quotations from Campbell are from this paper.

8. For a discussion of the problems blame can pose among those seeking to overcome their oppression see Sarah Hoagland (1988). For a response to her view see Houston (1992). In the *Hypatia* paper I argue in praise of blame. However, the context there concerns more personal relationships; and my argument is premised upon a Strawsonian notion of responsibility, a notion quite different from the modern concept of responsibility that lies at the heart of my arguments here.

9. Card is arguing that for those with diminished agency, it can be effective to focus on inner conflicts and inner resources and, if necessary, separation from those environments which induce a sense of powerlessness. She has in mind women who suffer from a childhood history of abuse or those who need to escape seriously subordinating conditions. She sees tak-

ing such measures as part of an integrity project. I am reluctant to join with her in seeing it as an integrity project primarily because I have reservations about her notion of integrity.

10. For a lucid discussion of Kierkegaard's notion of "double reflection" see Mark Dooley (2001).

11. My discussion of these risks has been shaped by conversations with Cynthia Cohen. See Cynthia Cohen, Working With Integrity: A Guidebook for Peacebuilders Asking Ethical Questions (Waltham, MA: The International Center for Ethics, Justice and Public Life, Brandeis University, 2001).

12. I am indebted to both Dwight Boyd (2003) and to Heesoon Bai (2003) for thoughtful commentary on an earlier version of this essay. They have each pointed out to me the necessity for carefully scrutinizing the assumptions about the self that underlie attributions of responsibility. While I cannot wholly adopt either of their pictures of the self, conversations with them have impressed upon me the need to better reconcile competing views if attributions of moral responsibility for systemic injustice are to be intelligible.

References

Bai, H. (2001). Cultivating democratic citizenship: Towards intersubjectivity. In W. Hare & J. P. Portelli (Eds.), *Philosophy of education: Introductory readings* (pp. 307-320). Calgary, AB: Detselig Enterprises Ltd.

Bai, H. (2003). Taking one's place in a moral universe. In S. Fletcher (Ed.), *Philosophy of education 2002* (pp. 19-22). Urbana, IL: Philosophy of Education Society.

Bartky, S. (2002). *Sympathy and solidarity and other essays.* New York: Rowman and Littlefield.

Berry, W. (1990). A poem of difficult hope. *What are people for?* New York: North Point Press.

Boler, M. (1999). *Feeling power: Emotions and education.* New York: Routledge.

Boyd, D. (1998). The place of locating oneself(ves)/myself(ves) in doing philosophy of education. In S. Laird (Ed.), *Philosophy of education 1997* (pp. 1-19). Urbana, IL: Philosophy of Education Society.

Boyd, D. (2003). Glass snakes vs groupals: Who is the responsible subject? In S. Fletcher (Ed.), *Philosophy of education 2002* (pp.14-18). Urbana, IL: Philosophy of Education Society.

Brandt, R. (1969). A utilitarian theory of excuses. *Philosophical Review 78,* 337-361.

Campbell, S. (2002). Emotion, memory and political identification. Paper presented to the Canadian Society for Women in Philosophy, The University of Guelph, Guelph, Ontario, Canada, September 2002.

Card, C. (1996). *The unnatural lottery.* Philadelphia: Temple University Press.

Cohen, C. (2001). *Working with integrity: A guidebook for peacebuilders asking ethical questions.* Waltham, MA: The International Center for Ethics, Justice and Public Life, Brandeis University.

Cousin, N. (2000). *Decent People.* Lanham, MD: Rowman and Littlefield.

deCastell, S. (This volume). No speech is free: Affirmative action and the politics of give and take.

Dooley, M. (2001). *The politics of exodus: Kierkegaard's ethics of responsibility.* New York: Fordham University Press.

Feinberg, J. (1968). Collective Responsibility. *Journal of Philosophy, 65*(21), 674-688.

Feinberg, J. (1970). *Doing and deserving.* Princeton, NJ: Princeton University Press.

Frankena, W. (1963). *Ethics.* Englewood Cliffs, NJ: Prentice Hall.

Frye, M. (1990). A response to *Lesbian ethics. Hypatia, 5*(3), 132-137.

Glover, J. (1970). *Responsibility*. London: Routledge and Kegan Paul.

Hoagland, S. (1988). *Lesbian ethics: Towards a new value*. Palo Alto, CA: Institute of Lesbian Studies.

Houston, B. (1992). In praise of blame. *Hypatia, 7*(4), 128–147.

Houston, B. (1994). Speaking candidly. In A. Thompson (Ed.), *Philosophy of education 1993* (pp. 110–113). Urbana, IL: Illinois State University Press.

Houston, B. (2003). Taking responsibility. In S. Fletcher (Ed.), *Philosophy of education 2002* (pp.1–13). Urbana, IL: Philosophy of Education Society.

Jones, A. (This volume). Talking cure: The impossibility of dialogue.

Kierkegaard, S. (1987). *Either/or* (H. Hong, Trans.). 2 Vols. Princeton: Princeton University Press.

Matsuda, M., C. Lawrence, R. Delgato, & K. Crenshaw (1993). *Words that wound*. Boulder, CO: Westview Press.

Noddings, N. (2002). *Educating moral people*. New York: Teachers College Press.

Rich, A. (1984). From an old house in America. *The fact of a doorframe*. New York: W. W. Norton.

Smart, J. J. C. (1961). Free will, praise and blame. *Mind, 70*, 291–306.

Smiley, M. (1992). *Moral responsibility and the boundaries of community*. Chicago: University of Chicago Press.

Strawson, P. F. (1974). *Freedom and resentment and other essays*. London: Methuen.

Walker, M. (1998). Moral understandings: A feminist study in ethics. New York: Routledge.

Williams, B. (1981). *Moral luck: Philosophical papers, 1973–1980*. Cambridge: Cambridge University Press.

Williams, P. (1997). *Seeing a color-blind future*. New York: Farrar, Straus and Giroux.

PART IV

Dialogue in Practice:
Risks and Benefits

Ann C. Berlak

Confrontation and Pedagogy: Cultural Secrets, Trauma, and Emotion in Antioppressive Pedagogies

How is it possible for many white students and students of color to be present in a university classroom where they read about, see videos documenting, and engage in activities that demonstrate the pervasive and ubiquitous realities and effects of institutional and personal racism, and yet fail to become engaged with racism at a deep emotional and analytical level? What can antiracist teachers do to promote engagement? The answers to these questions, I will argue, have less to do with ensuring opportunities for students from disempowered groups to speak, or for particular viewpoints to be spoken, than with trauma, erasure, mourning, and expression of feeling in classrooms.

The approach to antiracist teaching, and antioppression teaching more generally, that I develop in this essay emerged from an analysis of an encounter between an African American woman who made a guest presentation to a class I, a white woman, was teaching and the prospective and practicing teachers in the class. The presentation, much to the surprise of all of us, turned out to be traumatic for many students and evoked passionate feelings in virtually everyone present. After the students and I had reflected upon our responses to the encounter, our understanding of the power, ubiquity, and harm of racism and of our resistance to acknowledging it had grown exponentially.

What enabled students to begin to witness racism, or to deepen their abilities to witness it, I will argue, was the guest speaker's expression of anger in response to racism, which in turn aroused in students feelings that had previously been unrecognized, unspeakable, and unspoken. Furthermore, I will suggest that if a major purpose of teaching is to unsettle taken for granted views and feelings, then confrontation, with its attendant trauma, and reflection upon the trauma are necessary. Thus, confrontation and the intense emotional repercussions that are likely to follow may be essential to the process of eroding entrenched cultural acceptance of injustices such as racism. I will argue that "democratic dialogue" does not necessarily promote such shifts. I will, then, frame antioppression teaching as a route navigated between confrontation and reflection. Opportunities to navigate the route cannot be "planned" but may, as in this case, occur unpredictably.

Background: Teaching Before the Encounter

Since 1992 I have been exploring antiracist teaching in the context of teaching the state-mandated Cultural and Linguistic Diversity Course in the Department of Elementary Education at San Francisco State University. I have been teaching at a time when poor children and black and brown children of every social class, by virtually all indicators—grades, test scores, suspensions, and dropout and college attendance rates—continue to fall further behind white middle-class students with each additional year of schooling. The underachievement of African American students in particular is persistent and pervasive (Gay, 2001; Foster, 1996). The most frequent responses to these disparities have been more standardized and centralized testing, national standards, scripted curricula, vouchers, and privatization of schools. Rarely is it suggested that individual and institutional racism must be addressed if what is generally referred to as the achievement gap is to be reduced.[1]

Teaching this course for many years, reading the works of researchers such as King (1994) and Delpit (1997), and observing in classrooms have convinced me that racism does indeed contribute significantly to the gap.[2] However, very few students who arrive in my classroom are aware that racism is a major force in the society at large, much less that it is endemic to and perpetuated by schools.

My primary goal for the diversity course is to encourage students to rethink their assumptions about race, class, gender, culture, language, and sexual orientation that predispose them to reproduce rather than challenge injustice. I want them to recognize forms of injustice, including those that are least visible, and to become aware that as teachers they will have many opportunities to choose between collaborating with or challenging individuals and institutions that encourage indifference to oppression.

In the years that I have been promoting the unlearning of the "isms," I have looked most closely at racism. In the section of the course devoted to racism my goal is for students, both white and of color, to come to see themselves and others through the eyes of people whose positions in the racial hierarchy are different from their own. This includes seeing from the perspective of people of color who are attuned to the continuous mistreatment of people because of skin color and characteristics assumed to be associated with it. I also want students to become aware of the privileges white people enjoy just because of their whiteness if they have not already done so. Finally, I want the students to grasp racism deeply enough to be moved to interrupt it.

To promote these goals I ask students to write racial autobiographies investigating their induction into the racial hierarchy. We discuss videos that document institutional and personal racism, including *The Color of Fear,* in which a multiracial group of men express rage, anger, fear, and grief as they examine racism in their lives. We examine our reactions to James Baldwin's (1988) *A Talk to Teachers,* Gloria Yamato's (1998) *Something About the Subject Makes It Hard to Name,* and other essays that convey concretely and personally how the writers experience racism on a daily basis. We engage in class activities designed to raise awareness of white privilege and discuss current racial issues, including whether, as many initially believe, affirmative action gives unfair advantage to people of color. We consider how racism can breed internalized racism, the internalization or acceptance by people who are targets of racism of negative judgments made about them by society at large.[3]

We explore what a number of students think of as "reverse racism," a phrase that connotes to them the verbalization of antiwhite attitudes, and exclusion of white people from social events by people of color. I draw the distinction between the former and institutional racism, a term I use to refer to the systematic, naturalized and pervasive mistreatment and marginalization of, or violence against, a group of people on the basis of skin color. For the purposes of this course, I tell the students, the word *racism* will refer only to the latter. I make it clear that, given this definition of racism, "reverse racism" is a misleading and inaccurate term.

Students write responses to each class session, expressing their thoughts and feelings. I encourage candor by telling them I am looking for engagement with the issues rather than the degree to which their views are consonant with mine. I read and comment upon the journal entries and return them the following session.

Several years ago I had reached a point where I thought I had gone about as far as I could in designing a curriculum that would raise students' awareness of the ubiquity and severity of racism and internalized racism. Then the startling and surprising sequence of events that began with the encounter between the guest presenter, Sekani Moyenda, and my class occurred. The encounter and reflection upon it both revealed the limits of my teaching and deepened my understanding of antiracist pedagogy significantly. The efforts of Sekani and myself to understand what had happened suggested that the arousal and expression of passionate feelings and reflections upon that arousal and expression can provoke students to internalize information and perspectives regarding racism that had formerly fallen on deaf ears.

The Encounter and Its Aftermath

The events that impelled Sekani and me to rethink our understanding of antiracist pedagogy began on the July day when Sekani came to speak to the students in my diversity course.[4] Three quarters of the students in the course were of European descent. Most of the others were of Asian, Filipino, Latino/Latina, or mixed or biracial heritage. Only one was African American. Most of these students would be teaching in schools as racially and ethnically diverse as any in the world.[5]

Sekani is an African American woman who teaches at an elementary school in San Francisco that serves predominantly poor Chinese and African American families. She had been teaching with an emergency credential for several years and had been a student in the diversity course the previous semester. I invited her to speak because, after completing the course, she told me that, in her opinion, most graduates of teacher education programs were not prepared to deal with the realities they would face as teachers of African American, Latino, Asian immigrant, and poor children. She was convinced that many of those entering the profession were more likely to contribute to the destruction of these children than to their academic and personal growth and power.

The day before the presentation Sekani informed me she was going to engage the class in a simulation she had created to provoke thinking about classroom management in schools where most of the children are African American and poor. She planned to call the presentation "Boot Camp for Teachers." I had no idea what she had in store for us, though I knew for certain we would not be bored.

Sekani, arriving in African dress, introduced herself as someone who had grown up in the civil rights generation and, strongly influenced by her mother who had been a Black Panther, was a proponent of "I'm Black, I'm proud." She told the students she thought one of her primary functions as a teacher was to prepare children to become militant adults.

She then shared several autobiographical stories. One was a story of an experience she had when she was in fourth grade. During her first week at a new school where she was the only child of color, a white girl with "swooshing" long blond hair who sat in the desk in front of hers repeatedly annoyed her by swinging her hair on to Sekani's desk. Sekani expressed her annoyance several times to the girl and to the white teacher. Finally, after the teacher refused to intervene, she punched the girl. The girl arrived in school the next day with her hair pinned up "Heidi-style" and the harassment stopped.

After Sekani related this story, she posed the question, "What do you think I learned from this?" Several students suggested different possibilities, e.g., "You learned not to trust white people." Sekani responded, "That may have been what you would have learned. But the sense my child mind made of it was that a violent response can be an effective deterrent to those who insist on exploiting their white privilege."

The stories Sekani told conveyed that in her view racism profoundly and continuously affects her daily life and the lives of black, Asian, and Latino people, including the children the students in our class would be teaching. She stated explicitly that the most insidious forms of racism, in her opinion, are those that are unwittingly perpetrated by ordinary well-meaning people like themselves.

To provoke students to rethink their assumptions about classroom management in classrooms populated by poor black and Asian children she set up a "worst case scenario" role-play situation, which she called "credential students' greatest nightmare." It was a simulation of a fourth-grade classroom that had been taught by a succession of substitutes with emergency credentials. Most students were given scripts that described roles they were to play as children, paraprofessionals, or parents. Jim, a young white man, volunteered to be the teacher. There was immediate chaos as those assigned to be disruptive children fully embraced their disruptive roles. When faced with the simulated chaos, Jim called a "class meeting" to reiterate the class rules that Sekani had taped upon the wall. None of the "children" paid him any heed.

Jim became visibly agitated and red-faced. "Sit down," he yelled. "WE'RE HAVING A CLASS MEETING." After a few more minutes of chaos, the classroom a virtual madhouse, Sekani terminated the role-play.

Then, as I stood on the sidelines, Sekani conducted a twenty-minute debriefing of the role-play. Much of the debriefing was taken up by a heated exchange between Jim and Sekani that almost every student referred to that evening in their journals as an "argument." The argument included the following interchanges, spoken by both Sekani and Jim with increasingly passionate intensity:

JIM: "This situation is totally unrealistic. I've been teaching for a year and I've never seen it happen."

SEKANI: "Well I've seen it happen many times in the school where I teach. Especially in the classrooms of white teachers. It's based on my experience. I don't know where you've been teaching."

***

SEKANI: "What could you have done to diffuse the situation? Why didn't you use the 'para' to send the children who were out of control to the counselor?"

JIM: "I would never throw a child out of my classroom, no matter what. They'd never trust me if I did that."

SEKANI: "Perhaps knowing you will teach them what the limits are is just what they need in order to learn to trust you; abused and neglected children can't always be counted on to listen to reason."

***

At one point during the interchange between Jim and Sekani, Jim went over to the list of classroom rules Sekani had posted and below rule number eight he wrote number nine, "HAVE FUN" in bold letters. He told the class "I love being with kids. I'm just a kid, myself."

> SEKANI: "These children don't need an adult kid. They need adult role models; they can have fun *after* school. Your job is to teach. If you can't control the classroom, you can't teach. The children are there to learn. You better not sacrifice the learning of my children to what you think might be the needs of an out of control child. If you want to play, become a camp counselor."

Sekani said she could understand that some whites fear black children and adults. She told them she herself fears whites, particularly rednecks.

> JIM: "I don't appreciate your comments about rednecks; some of my best friends are rednecks."
> SEKANI: "Then you may want to reconsider working in a predominantly Black environment. None of us are too keen on YOUR friends."

Jim's and Sekani's voices had reverberated down the hall.

By the time the class period was over two of the white women in the class had shed tears, and one had fled the room before the class was over. I had remained silent on the periphery watching with amazement and awe as the confrontation unfurled. I recall wondering if an administrator would find out what had happened and question my judgment, or if, as a result of the frank and passionate expressions of feelings, students might report me to the Dean. However, what I remember most vividly was my stunned realization that, though we were nearing the conclusion of the course, we were just beginning to scratch the surface. I also realized that my surprise was an indication of how much I still had to learn.

Initial Responses to the Encounter: Denials and Affirmations of Sekani's Views

The students' journal entries written the night of the encounter indicated a number of them had questioned the validity of Sekani's views and interpretations, including her assumption that racism was a factor in the blond-haired girl story. I cite two examples. Jim wrote, "I don't think she [Sekani] is sensitive to the feelings of everyone. . . . It seems to me she is telling us 'the way it is' from a very one-sided point of view."

Kathy, a white sociology major who had an undergraduate degree from a high-status university, had previously written, in response to James Baldwin's essay, that she recognized the destructiveness of racism and was committed to becoming an antiracist teacher. The night of the encounter she wrote in her journal:

> I believe we have built a community based on our shared and differing experiences . . . and are respectful of what we have learned from each other and open to civil discussions of differing opinions. I found S . . . to be hostile, condemning and close minded . . . I found her attitude extremely condescending . . . I felt she completely dismissed any of our experiences . . . She claims she cannot be racist because she does not hold a position of power in society. When she entered our classroom, by taking on the role of teacher, she was in a position of power and she used that power to judge people and make disparaging comments on the basis of the color of their skin. Hmmmm. Sounds like RACISM to me.

It was not until I read this journal entry that I realized how superficial Kathy's earlier response to Baldwin's essay had been, and that she had not accepted the distinction I had drawn between racism and "reverse racism."

Prior to Sekani's visit Isaiah, the only African American in the class, had remained silent on issues related to race in the "open forums" of class discussions. Nor had he shared with me any concerns about expressions of racism in our class or elsewhere. The night of the encounter he wrote:

> Sekani touched a nerve in our classmates . . . She gave them more in two hours than they will get from any course or class at this university. She stated her agenda, and Jim and others attacked that agenda and forgot about the issue of teaching children of color. Our classmates should be grateful, not ANGRY. She opened or made people take their lenses off and LOOK! LOOK AT YOURSELF. LOOK AT YOUR STUDENTS. LOOK.

There were many more responses, including one by Jennifer, a white woman, who wrote,

> Whew!!! What a class!!! . . . The experience is probably the closest I have ever come to feeling like I know what I look like or could look like through the "lenses" of an African American woman. This information is so valuable to me . . . It was one of the most valuable classes I have ever had.

"Processing" the Encounter

In class the next day we spent an hour reflecting upon our reactions to the encounter. I organized the session by asking students to write answers to eight questions designed to elicit their thoughts and feelings about what had happened. I posed questions such as how they felt about the encounter, what they felt about Sekani's story of the blond-haired girl, what they thought Sekani wanted us to know about teaching, and whether I should invite her to present to future classes, and if so, what changes (if any) they thought she should make in her presentation.

After they had written responses to a question I asked each student to read his or her response to it aloud. My purpose was to provide the students with a sense of the variation in their classmates' thoughts and feelings. After the students had given their responses to a question I shared with them my own responses to it.

The following is a sample of journal entries students wrote the evening after the class session devoted to "processing" the encounter. Jim wrote,

> Today's class helped me to internalize the messages that were hard for me to grasp yesterday . . . I feel I'm really starting to GET IT. . . . What I'm starting to realize is that no matter what I feel, others have feelings and images that are just as real and also based on years of experience.

Isaiah wrote,

> . . . I really feel some of our classmates were intimidated by Sista Sekani . . . I'm really glad you did the [debriefing] exercise so the many emotions of our classmates could be heard. I know you would like me to speak up more when we have open discussions, but I don't believe our classmates can even hear ME . . . I feel totally shut out sometimes in our class and that may be ME trippin'. This is how I feel right now. ANGRY. I needed to know how people really see me . . . This class has been an awakening for me. I hope it awakens my fellow classmates. But my lenses have been opened as well.

Kathy wrote,

> I feel much better after today's class. I enjoyed the debriefing exercise. I had such a violent reaction after Tuesday's class I was unable to focus on any positive aspect of Sekani's presentation. After I had the experience of hearing other people's perspectives, I realized I had learned and gained more than I thought. It was good for me to hear her anger and examine the deep feelings it brought up for me.

Transformations

By the time the encounter and debriefing were completed a profound change had occurred in the tenor of the class. Whereas, before Sekani's visit, we had discussed racism in tones we might have used to talk about the weather, afterward virtually everyone was emotionally as well as analytically engaged. Sekani's visit had inadvertently unearthed residual veins of racism and provoked us as a class to confront them. It was an unanticipated happening that surprised us all.

By the end of the course there were indications the encounter and our reflections upon it had disturbed most students' anchoring worldviews and initiated some significant transformations. For example, after Sekani's visit Isaiah began to think about his feeling that his classmates could not hear him, and consider whether this feeling was the result of him "trippin.'" We might say he was beginning to see his and the white students' positions in the racial hierarchy through the eyes of James Baldwin, Sekani and myself. He was beginning to see himself as a black man who, in the words of Baldwin, had been "assured by his countrymen that he has never contributed anything to civilization." Furthermore, he was beginning to see his white classmates as people who, again in Baldwin's words, "try to deal with Negroes as though they were missionaries" (1988, pp. 7–9). He came to recognize that many of his classmates did not, in fact, hear him when he spoke. As he put it, "I needed to know how people see me . . . This class has been an awakening for me."

Jim's statement that he was "starting to realize . . . that . . . others have feelings and images that are just as real, and also based on years of experience" suggests a dawning awareness that Sekani, like himself, is a human being with "feelings and images." It also suggests it was occurring to him, perhaps for the first time, that Sekani had images *of him*, and that she might see him in ways that until that moment he had not seen himself. His statement could be taken as an expression of a nascent ability to receive information about how he might be seen and heard by others whose views he had been socialized to discount or not to hear at all.

Making Sense of the Encounter

How can a closer look at the encounter and its aftermath both help us understand the difficulty many students have acknowledging patterns of institutional and personal racism and shed light on how teachers can address this difficulty? My response to these questions draws upon several concepts from Shoshana Felman and Dori Laub's *Testimony*.

In *Testimony*, Felman and Laub investigate surviving victims', perpetrators', and bystanders' ways of responding to the unthinkable historical catastrophe of the extermination of nine million human beings by the Nazis. They sum up the views of many members of each of these groups toward the Holocaust as a great conspiracy of silence in which all parties collude, a great cultural secret we are all still keeping from ourselves (Felman & Laub, 1992, p. xix). Felman and Laub ask how it is possible for many of the victims, perpetrators, and bystanders to have been present at the atrocities and yet to have erased the events from consciousness, and consider the processes through which such secrets can be revealed.

I do not use the concepts from *Testimony* because I equate or compare present-day racism in the United States with the Holocaust. I use them because they helped me understand why it is so difficult for many students, both white and of color, to acknowledge the realities of racism, and also because they suggested ways of thinking about how teachers can provoke students' awareness of the shared cultural secret of institutional and personal racism.

Erasure

After reading *Testimony* I began to see racism as a cultural secret, that is, a phenomenon that is rarely felt, acknowledged, or spoken of in the dominant public discourse, in places of worship, the media, schools, and universities. The notion of cultural secret helped me bring into focus the fact that the vast majority of students in my credential classes, both white and of color, had never had a significant conversation about racism before they entered my classroom.

Felman and Laub use the concept *erasure* to refer to individuals' failures to perceive, recall, and respond with appropriate empathy to evidence of inhumane treatment that is, or has been, right before their eyes. They quote a man (speaking in the film *Shoah*) who had lived near a death camp to convey the quality of not-knowing of bystanders and perpetrators at the time: "It was always this peaceful here. Always. They burned two thousand people—Jews—every day . . . No one shouted. Everyone went about his work. It was silent. Peaceful. Just as it is now" (Felman & Laub, 1992, p. 259). This quote conveys erasure of mass murder from consciousness that for many, *Shoah* suggests, continues to the present day.

Felman and Laub's portrayals of erasure of the Holocaust by perpetrators and bystanders crystallized my awareness that many white and light-skinned students had remained impervious to evidence of racism they had been privy to both in and outside of class. I saw evidence of erasure in students' failures to suggest the possibility that racism might contribute to the racial achievement gap, even after they had been given many forms of evidence of the ubiquity of racism, including a video that compared experiences of a Black and a white man who apply for the same job, try to rent the same apartment, go shopping at the same stores, and encounter the same police. Another indication of erasure was some students' continuing tendencies to label accounts of racism "exaggeration" or "complaints."

Felman and Laub offer the voice of a lone survivor of one of the camps speaking in *Shoah* that clarified for me what it means to say that victims themselves often do not recognize or experience their own victimization. "When I saw all this, it didn't affect me . . . I was only thirteen and all I'd ever seen was dead bodies . . . I thought that was the way things had to be, that it was normal" (Felman & Laub, 1992, p. 258). Another, speaking of victims' blindness to the meaning of what they saw, describes a moment of perception coupled with incomprehension, an exemplary moment in which the Jews failed to read or decipher the visual sign they saw with their own eyes:

> "Then, very slowly, the train turned off the main track and rolled . . . through a wood. When he looked out . . . the window . . . the old man in our compartment saw a boy . . . and he asked the boy in signs, 'Where are we?' And the kid made a funny gesture, this." (He draws his finger across his throat.)
> "And one of you questioned him?"
> "Not in words, but in signs . . . We didn't really pay much attention to him. We couldn't figure out what he meant." (Felman & Laub, 1992, p. 208)

The claim by Isaiah that the encounter opened his eyes suggests that, prior to Sekani's visit, he, like many of his classmates, had also substantially erased racism from consciousness. Felman & Laub summarize, "To understand *Shoah* is to gain new insight into what not knowing means" (1992, p. 253).

Felman and Laub explain how it is possible for conscious beings to dismiss or erase the dehumanization of self and others. They see the failure of so many perpetrators, bystanders, and victims to grasp these events as a function of the fact that the events are "in excess of their frames of reference." That is, the victims, bystanders, and perpetrators do not have the languages, categories, or frameworks by which to name and categorize the events and cannot, therefore, assimilate them into full cognition (Felman, 1992, p. 5). Their preexisting culturally shared frames of reference both delimit and determine what they can know (1992, p. xv).

The substantial degree of erasure of racism by many students prior to and during most of the course can be understood as an effect of the limitations imposed by the frameworks or languages they had been immersed in since birth.[6] Their induction into the racial hierarchy began in early childhood when those on all sides of the racial divide were told or shown, implicitly and explicitly, that people with lighter skin are "more than"—more beautiful, more trustworthy, more intelligent, more civilized, and that the unequal treatment light and dark skinned people observe and receive is justified.[7] Though they initially resisted these messages, because children are relatively powerless in relationship to the adult world, for most institutionally racist interpretations and practices eventually became naturalized (Miller, 1983; Smith, 1961), as invisible as water to a fish. Though most of the students had forgotten the process through which their frameworks were forged, they lived inside them and were unable to register, and respond with appropriate feeling to, information that did not fit comfortably within them.

The frameworks constructed in childhood were reinforced and solidified by the media and schooling, both of which portrayed race relations as a story of continuous progress and treated the long histories of racism and antiracism in U.S. history superficially, if at all (Loewen, 1995). Thus, the media and schooling preserved the cultural secret of racism by minimizing its significance even as, with increasing subtlety, they portrayed race as a marker for inferiority/superiority (Sleeter, 1995). Psychology courses, central to teacher education programs, had focused students' attention almost entirely on individuals' abilities to shape their own destinies, thereby reinforcing worldviews that filtered out the effects of institutional racism. Therefore, most of the students had entered the classroom with lenses that could accommodate only a partial set of stories about the racial hierarchy, and the stories they could accommodate were partial to the powerful.[8]

The curriculum I had offered prior to Sekani's visit may be viewed as the presentation and exploration of evidence documenting some of the realities of racism through the use of video and print. Many students incorporated fragments of this evidence, and fewer students, both white and of color, continued to dismiss Baldwin's "complaints" as outdated, or expressed the thought that the men in *The Color of Fear* were "over-reacting" to racism. Students like Kathy, picking up on a metaphor I used regularly, began to write that they were refocusing their lenses, and beginning to recognize racism and even to speak out against it. However, I doubt anyone had developed a deep and coherent awareness of racism. Breaking through the erasures and becoming witnesses to racism awaited the expression of passionate feelings that characterized the encounter.

Trauma and Witnessing

Two additional concepts offered by Felman and Laub, *trauma* and *witnessing,* helped me understand more about the dynamics behind the transformations. In Felman and Laub's view, one function of the frameworks that filter experience is to protect us from awareness of painful events. Trauma, as I use it here, refers both to massive, painful, isolated events outside the normal range of human experience and to daily insidious and persistent events that continue to re-injure the wounded (see Erickson, this volume). What distinguishes traumatic events from other injurious events is their effects: The traumatic event or pattern of events and/or the feelings aroused by them (Herman, 1992) are initially partially or wholly erased from consciousness (Britzman, 2000).[9]

Many of the injuries racism inflicts on people of color are more easily identified than those it inflicts on white people. Racism does, however, also injure white people. A primary way it does so is by separating them from their humanity as moral beings. Lillian Smith, a white woman writing in the pre–Civil Rights Era South provides an example of the traumatic injury racism can cause white people when she writes of being repeatedly told as a child that the love and tenderness she received from and felt toward her black nurse was a childish thing she must outgrow, and that, more generally, the human relations she valued most were of little value in the world in which she lived (1961, p. 29). She says, "We learned the dance that cripples the human spirit step by step by step" (1961, p. 96).

Smith shows how repressing significant elements of one's moral being severs connections between cognition and feeling, and "numbs" white people to injustices. Such numbing can be so wide-ranging and persistent that it comes to be taken as an enduring characteristic of one's personality or culture (Herman, 1992, p. 48). This process of becoming numb is then "forgotten." In Smith's words, "The ceremonials in honor of white supremacy, performed from babyhood, slip from the conscious mind deep down into muscles and glands" (1961, p. 96).

To gain cognitive and emotional awareness of, or have a visceral encounter with, trauma is to become a witness to it (Felman & Laub, 1992, p. 114). Because trauma cannot be contained within the schemas through which potential witnesses habitually receive information about their world, witnessing requires the destruction of taken for granted categories or frames of reference and the construction of new ones. This is a complex process that usually requires the help of another as shall be considered in more detail below.

Becoming a witness to traumatic events can be doubly painful. First, the shattering of naturalized worldviews is profoundly disorienting and painful in itself. Second, witnessing experiences that had previously been filtered out is painful because what enters consciousness through the transformed frameworks is itself painful and terrifying. Thus, say Felman and Laub, the witness "becomes radically transformed by the very process of witnessing" (1992, p. 10).

Witnessing can be firsthand, that is, the victims—those who are directly confronted by a traumatic event or daily persistent injuries—come to a deep awareness of the dehumanizing events they have experienced but erased. Because induction into the racial hierarchy has been traumatizing to them, white people as well as people of color are potential firsthand witnesses to trauma caused by racism.

White people can also become secondhand witnesses to racism. Through secondhand witnessing a perpetrator or bystander becomes imaginatively capable of perceiving and feeling the victims' trauma in his or her own body—gaining "the power of sight (or insight) usually afforded only by one's own immediate physical involvement" (Felman & Laub, 1992, p. 108).[10] Becoming a secondhand witness to racism—imagining victims' trauma in their own bodies—is painful for second-hand witnesses because, as for the victims themselves, it involves shattering frameworks and integrating painful knowledge.

Trauma, Witnessing, and Mourning in the Classroom

Why did the encounter and debriefing provoke changes in consciousness that my entire curriculum until that point in time had not? What did it take for students to become first- or secondhand witnesses to racism? First, the traumatizing emotional power of the face-to-face encounter set the stage for transformations in both first- and secondhand potential witnesses. Second, both first- and secondhand potential witnesses' responses to the trauma were received and heard empathetically by the teacher and others in the class. Being listened to and heard enabled some to begin or to continue a process of mourning that made it possible to witness and integrate the trauma evoked and/or restimulated by the encounter. I will consider trauma, witnessing, and mourning as they occurred in our classroom in more detail below.

Trauma in the Classroom

When Sekani confronted Jim during the post-role-play "argument," many who had remained silent, as indicated in their journals, felt Jim had been speaking for them. They therefore felt Sekani's passionate challenge to Jim was also aimed directly at them and were, like Jim, initially, unable to integrate what she was saying into their worldviews. Thus, the encounter was a traumatic experience for many students.

Many must have experienced her challenge as particularly assaultive because it came from a black female. The frameworks through which most of them made sense of the world took as given that a black woman's ideas about how to be an effective teacher of black children and children of Asian heritage should not be taken as more authoritative than those of a white man, or indeed, any light skinned person of either gender. Tim, a Chinese immigrant from Hong Kong and Daren, a white male, suggest this interpretation. Tim: "The 'white' [students] probably felt more hurt since the comment came from a black female teacher who might unconsciously be considered to be not that intelligent." Daren: "A dynamic (that I absolutely will not bring up in class) is that Jim was not prepared to accept . . . critique from an African American woman, especially one as strong and militant as today's speaker."

What is more, many must have believed I was also challenging their worldviews because I remained silent and allowed the encounter to continue. One white woman wrote, "As a guest her opinions are validated . . . that alarms me . . . I wondered why you didn't intervene." She was expressing the expectation that I as a white woman would protect students from such challenges.

Many students were traumatized by the encounter simply because Sekani challenged assumptions about racial hierarchy that, as I argue below, were fundamental to their conceptions of self. However, the challenge was especially traumatizing because Sekani delivered it in tones that broke the norm against expressing emotion in classrooms. Her call to the students went beyond the expression of anger. She expressed rage. Her rage conveyed that racism is an assault upon her soul and upon the very nature or her people. It sent the message that racism is a wound that can not be healed unless fundamental and lasting change occurs—unless whites and white-dominated institutions become so fundamentally changed as to be unrecognizable.[11] This message was almost certainly in excess of every student's frame of reference.

Sekani's breaking the norm against expressing feeling in classrooms appeared to give permission to students to recognize and express *their* feelings. Indications of this include Jim's red face, the loud intense exchanges between him and Sekani, an explosive retort by Kathy to Sekani, and the tears of two white women, as well many references to fear and anger in their journals. One white woman wrote in her final journal entry:

> I feel like my insides have been ripped out and been replaced . . . So far this has been my range of emotions: intimidation, fear, defensive attitude, hopelessness, realization, guilt, confusion, hope, understanding, admiration, respect. And I would say that's just the tip of the iceberg.

Recall Isaiah's words, written the evening following the encounter, "This is how I feel right now. ANGRY." In all my many years of teaching, my students' feelings had never been activated as powerfully as they were by the encounter with Sekani.

Sekani had challenged the students to see themselves as people who had internalized racist messages, erased those messages and their significance from consciousness, and, usually without their awareness, acted upon them. This provocation activated feelings of anger, fear, and shame. Whereas Isaiah's anger was what Megan Boler (1999) refers to as moral anger, anger at socially induced suffering, the anger many of the students expressed during and after the encounter, initially, at least, was of another kind—what Boler calls defensive anger. Defensive anger can be a response to shame induced by the belief one is being blamed for the injustices that provoked the moral anger. Defensive anger can also be a defense against fear.

Prior to Sekani's visit, no student had expressed any fears to me or to the class. After Sekani's visit there were many expressions of fear. One white female student wrote of the post-role-play interchanges between Jim and Sekani: "The discussion became invasive, violent." Another wrote, "When she [Sekani] explained that her goal as a teacher was to bring up militant boys and girls . . . off the top of my head I associated it with words like military and war." Another claimed to have heard "our speaker mention the word 'militarism.'" A student wrote that her heart rate increased in response to the questions I posed during the processing session. Why had my asking questions caused her heartbeat to quicken? What did she fear?

Sekani's expression of anger and rage, her references to "militancy," and her story of the blond-haired girl, likely restimulated fears of black violence that had originally accompanied most students' induction into the racial hierarchy. Given the frequency of media portrayals of crime and violence perpetrated by black men, the role-play likely evoked terror at the prospect of dealing with what many had learned to see as violence-prone black children and their parents.

Jim's interchange with Sekani about "rednecks" may have provoked in him and others the fear that if they began to see racism from Sekani's point of view, they would be setting themselves apart from their families or friends. Fears of not belonging reside in the most vulnerable corners of our psyches. Perhaps at least some of the students, though they were unaware of it, were deeply invested in keeping at bay Sekani's view that she and other people of color had been unjustly disempowered, because they feared destruction of fundamental beliefs about how rewards and punishments are meted out in a society they had learned to think of as just.

Some of the students' defensive anger may have also served as a shield against recognizing that their moral compasses were failing them. Some of the white and light-skinned students who responded with defensive anger may have been resisting facing the shameful awareness that they had in fact been bystanders to racism—that they had not noticed, and were not outraged or even moved by, injustices experienced by others. Shame, in contrast to guilt, is a self-judgment not against one's acts, but upon one's very being. Their shame regarding their failure to become outraged by racism may have been intimately connected with a profound desire to be recognized as worthy of respect. Maybe Jim's and other students' defensive anger was a response to a dawning awareness that their positions in the racial hierarchy, which provided important sources of self-esteem, might be unearned and undeserved.

Mourning: Becoming Witnesses by Being Heard

The encounter initially provoked erasure of Sekani's message, for example Kathy's and Jim's failure to take seriously Sekani's testimony that racism affected her daily experience, and Isaiah's continuing difficulty acknowledging racism. ("That may be me trippin.") It also evoked strong, and, for most, aversive, feelings without suggesting any way to adequately respond to them.[12] For many, this aroused anxiety—a generalized feeling of dread.

However, though an unpleasant sensation, anxiety can set the stage for a moment of transformation in those who have the spirit and inclination to recognize and reflect upon their emotional responses and go beyond them. In fact, trauma, defensive and moral anger, and anxiety can be seen as essential precursors to the complex dynamic involved in mourning.[13] Mourning is a process of naming and confronting one's own and others' suffering, of recognizing and coming to terms with loss, whether the loss be of an actual person, a way of making sense of social experience, or an ideal (Britzman, 2000). It can free those who experience it to participate energetically in unraveling the institutional structures that keep injustices in place.

Mourning is set in motion when one begins to reflect upon trauma one has experienced. It is this form of self-reflection that Jim expressed after the processing session when he wrote, "While the role play exercise was in progress . . . I was angered and defensive." Kathy reflected upon her initial reaction to the encounter by writing, "I had such a violent reaction after Tuesday's class. I think it was good for me to hear her anger and to examine the deep feelings it brought up for me."

How is it possible to mourn the various losses incurred by one's own and others' racism, in the face of a psychological and cultural dynamic that militates against acknowledging such suffering in oneself and others? Felman & Laub (1992) suggest that it is being heard empathetically that enables individuals to become witnesses to trauma they have experienced and to traumatic experiences of others. In their words, "It takes two to witness the unconscious" (p. 115).

Individuals can not empathize with the pain of others if they have not brought to consciousness and experienced the pain they themselves have been directly subjected to (Miller, 1983). Thus, the trauma white people experienced as they were socialized into the racial order must be heard empathetically if they are to become secondhand witnesses to the trauma people of color experience firsthand.

Being an empathetic listener requires having mourned enough of one's own traumatic experience to be able to hear and respond empathetically to, rather than erase, what potential witnesses are saying. To "hear" the trauma of another, listeners must have the frameworks and categories that enable them to apprehend the clues the potential witness offers to what he or she grasps only dimly if at all. Hearing is made more difficult because people who have experienced trauma often prefer to remain silent in order to protect themselves from the fear of being heard and thus of hearing themselves (Felman & Laub, 1992, p. 58). Responding empathetically involves conveying that failure to feel and know one's own pain and the pain of others is a consequence of social experience and, therefore, has been, for the most part, beyond conscious control.

Students' Experiences of Being Listened to and Being Heard

After the encounter students had several opportunities for feelings that had been evoked by the trauma of the encounter to be listened to with empathy and heard, by their classmates and by me. During the processing session, as they read aloud and listened to responses to my questions about the traumatic experiences they had shared, they discovered there was at least one other student who shared their views and feelings. Thus, during the processing session, everyone had the opportunity to have his or her feelings heard by an empathetic other. Students had "the right to pass," but on the day we reflected together upon Sekani's visit everyone seemed eager to share at least some of their feelings and views. The debriefing session also revealed that refusal to acknowledge the validity of Sekani's concerns and feelings was not the only response possible. It therefore put students who had continued to erase Sekani's perspectives in a position to reflect further upon their own feelings and views.

Felman (1992) describes her students' delayed reactions to testimonies of Holocaust survivors, perpetrators, and bystanders that resulted in part from intense interactions with one another outside of class. Such interactions were another venue where students' feelings could be heard empathetically. The journals of my students document a similar process that likely contributed to their changing views.

I also listened with empathy to the students' responses to the trauma that was provoked or re-evoked by the encounter. I communicated my empathetic understanding both during the processing session and in my written responses to the journals. (In fact, throughout the course I had, in my responses to journal entries, "heard" and encouraged students to acknowledge the pain they had experienced as a result of being subjected to any of the " isms," including adultism.)

I could listen with empathy because I myself had previously been listened to with empathy as I grappled with my own defensiveness and erasures, and could therefore understand from personal experience and convey to students that their erasures of racism and their defensive anger resulted from their socialization and had been beyond their control. I could also convey that their fear, anxiety, and shame could be seen as initial stages in the process of becoming witnesses to racism.

During the course I made no special effort to provide Isaiah with an opportunity to speak to his classmates, many of whom he correctly suspected would not in any case have heard him. By inviting Sekani what I did provide him was an expression of rage by another who shared his experience of being targeted by racism. Although he did not speak directly to her, Sekani played the role of empathetic listener for Isaiah by affirming his reality and the legitimacy of his latent rage.[14]

The work we had done in class before Sekani's visit, and the work some students had done before the course began, had prepared some to begin to recognize and mourn the cruelty, fear, and shame incurred by racism, and to consider the gains that confronting racism in ourselves and in society makes possible. For others, the mobilization of fear, shame, anxiety, and resistance that are the prerequisites to mourning began only on the day Sekani entered our classroom.

For some, the opportunity to catch a glimpse of how Sekani saw and felt about them, traumatic though it was, became the most powerful and significant experience they had ever had in a classroom. This was as true for Isaiah as it was for Jennifer. Why would this be so? Perhaps because, by showing them how they looked to her, Sekani was revealing to them aspects of themselves they had been struggling to shut out. The recovery of those denied aspects of themselves may have increased their sense of wholeness and may therefore explain why so many were so enlivened by the encounter and our subsequent reflection upon it.

Lessons from the Encounter: Disturbing and Affirming Silenced Feelings

Megan Boler, in the conclusion to *Feeling Power,* states, "The best antiracist . . . work I have studied and seen in action is not about confrontation but rather a mutual exploration" (1999, p. 199). I would have agreed with this before Sekani and I began to revisit and examine the encounter and its aftermath. However, I now believe that if a major purpose of teaching is the promotion of students' abilities to receive information that is dissonant, not just congruent, with what they have learned before, then confrontation with its attendant trauma is necessary. I have come to concur with Felman and Laub that crisis is essential in order for cultural secrets to be revealed.

However, though many students in our class were only able to grapple with racism at a deep emotional and cognitive level because the encounter with Sekani had been traumatizing for them, speaking their feelings about the experiences they had shared and having their responses to it heard was also necessary. The artistry of teaching might then be seen as artful navigation between exploration and confrontation.

What happened in class was not the result of a deliberate strategy to provoke a crisis (see Erickson, this volume), but an accident. The process was set in motion when I invited a guest into the classroom who was willing to express with passion insurrectionist views that challenged students' frameworks for making sense of their social worlds. As Alison Jones argues (this volume), it is not the responsibility of marginalized or colonized students to fulfill this educative role; in fact, teachers are responsible for constructing a curriculum that is as educative for marginalized as for more privileged students.

The encounter was an extraordinary event. What conclusions can we draw from it that can inform our practice on those many "ordinary" teaching days? What I have come to understand from teaching since the encounter is that it is not necessary to initiate a process of exploding cultural secrets by inviting a guest to class. I have become increasingly aware that whenever racism or any other cultural secret is the topic of discussion trauma, in one guise or another, is also present, an ubiquitous, but most frequently unrecognized and uninvited guest. We simply need to recognize the clues to its presence, the courage to acknowledge and explore the disturbing feelings it evokes, and the willingness to support students in mourning the pain that bursting open cultural secrets entails. If we do not recognize the presence of trauma and welcome and reflect upon it, we insure that students will be left in harmful repetitions that reproduce the status quo.

Much of what is taken to be "democratic dialogue" is a repetition that does not disrupt the common wisdom. That my pedagogy had at best been marginally disruptive prior to Sekani's visit was powerfully revealed on the day she came to class. The failure to recognize and honor troubling feelings in our classrooms sustains cultural secrets. It permits students to remain comfortable by reading stories of oppression and injustice as exaggerations and exceptions, and narratives of justice as the rule.

Notes

I want to acknowledge Megan Boler for her patience and invaluable feedback, Elsa Johnson for her clarification of several key ideas, and Harold Berlak for his support and editorial and substantive contributions.

1. See, for example, a story by Viadero (2000) on the front page of the "mainstream" education periodical *Education Week* entitled, "Lags in Minority Achievement Defy Traditional Explanations." Though in this essay I will speak of racism in the singular, I want to acknowledge that there are many forms of racism, and the processes the term refers to change over time. All forms, however, are maintained by institutional power.

2. An interrelated but also independent factor is, of course, institutionalized social class injustice, or inequalities of wealth.

3. See Carter (1995) for an analysis of the dangers of assuming that racism is necessarily internalized by people of color. Some may internalize racism; others develop appropriate anger in response to it. Many respond in both of these ways.

4. This account and analysis of the encounter is adapted from Ann Berlak and Sekani Moyenda (2001) *Taking It Personally: Racism in Classrooms from Kindergarten to College.*

5. In California 60% of public school students and fewer than 23% of their teachers are persons of color (Keheler et al., 1999, p. 10).

   Each of the classes depicted in *Troubling Speech* has a unique racial (and class and gender) composition and geographical and historical location, and these are central to each analysis. In the classes I have taught at San Francisco State no student has ever made the case for the protection of hate speech.

6. White foreign students from Spain and France, like U.S. students, are usually unaware of racism in their countries of origin.

7. In a remarkable study of preschoolers Debra Van Ausdale (2001) shows how early the process of racist conditioning begins. Three of the best explications of this process I know of are Lillian Smith's, *Killers of the Dream* (1961), Minnie Bruce Pratt's "Identity: Skin/Blood/Heart" (1984) and Alice Miller's *For Your Own Good* (1983).

8. See Kumashiro (2001) for an extended exploration of these related meanings of "partial" in relationship to antioppressive education.

9. Forms and degrees of trauma vary and there is no "essential" form. Herman writes of trauma, "Traumatic reactions occur when . . . neither resistance nor escape is possible (and) the human system of self defense becomes overwhelmed . . . The traumatized person may experience intense emotion but without clear memory of the event, or may remember everything in detail but without emotion" (1992, p. 34).

10. A number of scholars have examined what Megan Boler (1999) calls the risks of empathy. One major concern is that an empathetic person may reduce the pain another feels to what she herself feels, wiping out the difference in circumstances, thinking, "Her pain is just like mine," rather than "my pain is like hers in this one way" (Berlak & Moyenda, 2001). Of course, secondhand witnesses can never gain a complete grasp of victims' traumas, and it is important that they understand the differences between first- and secondhand witnessing.

11. Kohl (2003). Kohl refers to Frantz Fanon's *Wretched of the Earth* (1986) for his analysis of rage. Felman describes a similar trauma that occurred after she showed her class videos of testimonies by Holocaust survivors. She wrote, "The class felt actively addressed not only by the video, but by the intensity and intimacy of the testimonial encounter throughout the course (p. 48). I see the face-to-face encounter with Sekani as even more intense and intimate than testimony given by video, in our case, the video, *The Color of Fear*.

12. The analysis that follows depends heavily upon Salverson (2000).

13. According to Felman & Laub (1992), "Innocence can only mean lack of awareness . . . guilt is not a state opposed to innocence; it is a process of awakening" (p. 196). Here Felman using the term *guilt* for what I understand as shame.

14. Isaiah did not leave the class with undirected anger. In a final project he wrote, "Finally, my goal for Sam (a student he had interviewed) is to be a "soldier," NOT a ghetto soldier but a soldier (who will). . .fight the injustices of people who are racist . . . (M)y agenda is to teach a little soldier who will be smart, real tough (physically and mentally) and educated."

References

Baldwin, J. (1988). A talk to teachers. In R. Simonson and S. Walker (Eds.), *The graywolf annual five: Multicultural literacy*. St. Paul, MN: Greywolf. (Original work published in 1963)

Berlak, A., & S. Moyenda. (2001). *Taking it personally: Racism in classrooms from kindergarten to college*. Philadelphia, PA: Temple University Press.

Britzman, D. (2000). If the story can not end: Deferred action, ambivalence and difficult knowledge." In R. Simon, S. Rosenberg, and C. Eppert (Eds.), *Beyond hope and despair: Pedagogy and the representation of historical trauma*. Totowa, NJ: Rowman and Littlefield.

Boler, M. (1999). *Feeling power: Emotions and education*. New York: Routledge.

Carter, R. (1995). *The influence of race and racial identity in the psychotherapy process: Towards a racially inclusive model*. New York: Wiley.

Delpit, L. (1997). *Other people's children: Cultural conflict in the classroom*. New York: The New Press.

Erickson, I. (This volume). Fighting fire with fire: Jane Elliot's antiracist pedagogy.

Felman, S., & D. Laub. (1992). *Testimony: Crises of witnessing in literature and psychoanalysis.* New York: Routledge.

Foster, M. (1996). As California goes, so goes the nation. *Journal of Negro Education, 65*(2), 105–111.

Gay, G. (2001). Educational equality for students of color. In J. Banks & C. Banks (Eds.), *Multicultural education.* New York: Wiley.

Herman, J. (1992). *Trauma and recovery.* USA: Basic Books.

Jones, A. (This volume). Talking cure: The desire for dialogue.

Keleher, T. (1999). *Creating crisis: How California teaching policies aggravate racial inequalities in public schools.* Oakland: Applied Research Center.

King, J. (1994). "The purpose of schooling for African American children: Including cultural knowledge." In E. Hollins, J. King, & W. Hayman (Eds.), *Teaching diverse populations: Formulating a knowledge base.* Albany: State University of New York Press.

Kohl, H. (2003). The fire this time: A review of *Taking it personally* by Ann Berlak and Sekani Moyenda. *Social Education.*

Kumashiro, K. (2001). "Posts" perspectives on antioppressive education in social studies, English, mathematics, and science classrooms. *Educational Researcher, 30* (3), 3–12.

Loewen, J. (1995). *Lies my teacher told me.* New York: Touchstone.

Mun Wah, L. Producer. (1994). *The color of fear.* Berkeley: Stir Fry Productions.

Miller, A. (1983). *For your own good: Hidden cruelty in child rearing and the roots of violence.* New York: Farrar, Straus & Giroux,.

Pratt, M. B. (1984). Identity: Skin, blood/heart. In E. Bulkin, et al. (Eds.), *Yours in struggle.* New York: Longhaul Press.

Salverson, J. (2000). Anxiety and contact in attending to a play about landmines. In R. Simon, S. Rosenberg, & C. Eppert (Eds.), *Between hope and despair: Pedagogy and the representation of historical trauma.* Totowa, NJ: Rutgers University Press.

Sleeter, C. (1995). Reflections on my use of multicultural and critical pedagogy when students are white. In C. Sleeter & P. McLaren (Eds.), *Multicultural education, critical pedagogy and the politics of difference.* Albany, NY: State University of New York Press.

Smith, L. (1961). *Killers of the dream.* New York: Norton. (Original work published in 1949)

Van Ausdale, D., & J. Feagin. (2001). *The first R: How children learn race and racism.* Rowman and Littlefield.

Viadero, D. (March 22, 2000). Lags in minority achievement defy traditional explanations. *Education Week.*

Yamato, G. (1998). Something about the subject makes it hard to name. In M. Anderson & P. Collins (Eds.), *Race, class and gender* (pp. 89–94). New York: Wadsworth.

Ingrid M. Erickson

Fighting Fire with Fire: Jane Elliott's Antiracist Pedagogy

In 1968, following the assassination of the Reverend Dr. Martin Luther King, Jr., Riceville, Iowa, schoolteacher Jane Elliott developed an exercise called "Blue Eyes, Brown Eyes" to teach her white, Christian, third-grade pupils about discrimination. She divided her students into two groups based on eye color, telling them that the brown-eyed students were superior—smarter, more responsible, and harder working than the blue-eyed children. The blue-eyed children, Elliott told them, were lazy, slow to learn, and not to be trusted. She withdrew the blue-eyed children's basic classroom rights, such as drinking directly from the water fountain. Brown-eyed children were moved up to the front of the class and granted special privileges. They were allowed to take extra time at recess, seconds at lunch, and so forth. Elliott fastened strips of cloth as collars around the necks of the blue-eyed children. Throughout the day, Elliott was quick to point out the shortcomings of the blue-eyed children, while lavishing praise on the favored group. Elliot was shocked to see how quickly her students were transformed—the blue-eyed children became frightened, timid, and uncertain, while the brown-eyed children excelled academically and quickly became arrogant, domineering, and overbearing. On the second day of the exercise, Elliott reversed the order, making the blue-eyed children superior, with the same results. Elliott had told the children it was all right to judge each other based on their eye color, but she did not have to teach them how to oppress each other. The conclusion Elliott drew from her exercise was that racism is learned. Racism could be created, and, as she says, "as with anything, if you can create it, you can destroy it."

In 1970, ABC produced a documentary about Elliott's classroom exercise entitled *The Eye of the Storm*. This video has been widely used in teacher preparation to demonstrate the pernicious effects of discrimination on student performance. Elliott continued to do her antidiscrimination exercise through the next sixteen years in her Riceville classroom. In 1986, Elliott retired from her teaching position to do antiracist work among adults in universities, the public sector, and the corporate setting.

Still today, Elliott repeats her Riceville classroom experience in her work with adults, but she does so in ways that are, as she puts it in a recent (2001) video, *The College Eye,* "mean and nasty." Her goal is to "inoculate" her participants against prejudice. In promotional materials for *The College Eye,* Elliott says: "I consider this exercise an injection of the live virus of racism." Since most people of color have brown eyes, Elliott designates the blue-eyed participants as the inferior group. To administer this virus, Elliott subjects her blue-eyed participants to discrimination. She badgers, humiliates, and insults them, repeatedly reminding them that their suffering is nothing compared to the daily experiences of people of color within American culture. Elliott is much more direct with her adult participants than she was with her grade school pupils. Stifling all attempts to object or engage in discussion, she silences her participants as people in American culture are silenced because of their skin color. Elliott's workshops are both painful and powerful, and her work is in many ways highly effective in addressing skin-color privilege and prejudice.

Elliott is certainly among the best known "crusaders" against racism in our times. Since her first appearance on the Tonight Show with Johnny Carson, Elliott has been a guest on Donahue, ABC News, PBS Frontline, 60 Minutes, and in 1992 on the Oprah Winfrey Show. Elliott's work on Oprah was rebroadcast in 2002. She was ABC's Person of the Week with Peter Jennings, and has been awarded the National Mental Health Association Award for Excellence in Education. Elliott's award-winning videos[1] are widely used in diversity training and teacher education, and she commands high consulting fees to present her workshops in businesses, public schools, and prisons.

Despite a long and successful history of work against racism and discrimination, a closer look at Elliott's strategies reveals a number of paradoxes. Elliott models behavior she hopes to eliminate, challenges privilege using the tools that have been traditionally used by those in power, and in general employs a range of pedagogical methods many progressive educators would shun. Elliott's medical metaphors rely on an essentialist discourse of race, one that simplifies the complex histories of racism in the name of certainty. Indeed, it may be argued that Elliott's effectiveness as a trainer depends on such a discourse. A closer investigation of the paradox implicit in Elliott's attempts to challenge power and privilege through its blatant use in the training setting may yield some insight into the ethical dilemmas posed by such practices. Locating Elliott's work within two frameworks—current theories on trauma and the affirmative action pedagogy proposed by Megan Boler in this volume—this essay explores some of the paradoxes involved in using silencing as a strategy.

This essay is part of a larger project exploring the relationship between trauma and learning. For the past six years, I have provided training in diversity and cultural competence within the University of Wisconsin-Milwaukee community. Diversity training inevitably involves trauma, as participants' beliefs and views are challenged and their sense of themselves as moral beings is unsettled by an encounter with the workings of power and privilege. As a diversity trainer, I am always searching for methods to provoke a confrontation with injustice and privilege—methods that will necessarily be painful but that will not inflict lasting harm on participants. I often find myself wondering how much trauma is enough, how much is too much, and whether I have the facilitation skills adequate to bring a group back from trauma so that they can learn from the experience. I came into contact with Jane Elliott's methods and with her reputation as a trainer early in my own diversity work. I continue to find myself troubled by certain aspects of Elliott's work, while at the same time, I am increasingly skeptical about how much learning takes place in classroom settings where trauma does not occur. I am also suspicious of my own resistance to inflicting trauma, because, as a white person, I have largely been able to avoid trauma in ways that my colleagues of color have not. I believe that my resistance to Elliott's methods mirrors the ambiguity and discomfort experienced by many educators who recognize the need to provoke deep and often painful reflection at the same time that they resist the need to induce trauma. If responsible educators are indeed compelled to induce trauma by challenging certain beliefs because they are wrong or destructive to self or other, then we may inevitably find ourselves in a judgmental and dogmatic position that may be quite uncomfortable for us to occupy. However, it seems clear that little learning about privilege and discrimination takes place in a learning environment that is free of trauma, and also that a lapse into a position of moral relativism is an unacceptable alternative. This essay will use Elliott's work to explore these and related tensions.

In her recent work on psychoanalysis and learning, Deborah Britzman poses the following challenge to educators:

> For, if education must interfere with psychic and social development, with the pushes and pulls of superstitious and stereotypical thought, and with a narcissism that so easily becomes attached to and defended by all sorts of prejudices, then how does education decide which force of interference shall matter? How can education recognize and repair not just the harm done by others but the harm that occurs under the name of education? How can education recognize and repair its own harm? (Britzman, 1998, p. 9)

In the diversity training setting, the type of interference Britzman refers to is foundational, and takes the form of challenging the beliefs and assumptions of session participants. It can be argued that only such a traumatic challenge will awaken an awareness of unearned privilege, that nothing but discomfort will provoke the self reflection needed to understand one's relationship to those who are different from oneself and the often painful knowledge of complicity with oppressive power structures that entails.

Trauma Theory

Let me set the stage for this discussion by clarifying my use of the term "trauma." In its original formulation, trauma referred to a blow or a wound, or more precisely, to the aftermath of such a blow. Dominic LaCapra refers to trauma as "a shattering break or cesura in experience which has belated effects" (2001, p. 186). The *Comprehensive Textbook of Psychiatry* defines the common reaction to trauma as "intense fear, helplessness, loss of control, and threat of annihilation" (cited in Herman, 1997, p. 11). Trauma theory has had a peculiar history, beginning at the turn of the last century with the work of Charcot and Janet in France, Freud and Breuer in Austria, re-emerging after the First World War and again after the Vietnam War with work on "shell-shocked" veterans, and again in the twentieth century with discussions of sexual and domestic trauma. Judith Herman (1997) describes a curious history of "episodic amnesia" (p. 7) in the field of trauma theory, alternating periods of active investigation with periods of oblivion. Herman links phases of active interest in trauma with political movements, describing, for instance, how the growth of an anti-war movement provided the political context for the study of shell shock or combat neurosis, while the feminist movement in Western Europe and North America provided a political context for an examination of the trauma resulting from sexual and domestic violence (1997, p. 9). Ruth Leys also describes the waxing and waning of interest in trauma, noting that it was essentially a political struggle to acknowledge the postwar suffering of Vietnam veterans that finally brought official recognition of Posttraumatic Stress Disorder in the third version of the American Psychiatric Association's Diagnostic and Statistical Manual of Mental Disorders, published in 1980 (Leys, 2000).

The Diagnostic and Statistical Manual (DSM), the so-called diagnostic "bible" of practitioners of therapy, is used to assess whether a diagnosis of trauma is warranted. Only since the 1994 publication of the DSM IV has the definition of posttraumatic stress been expanded to include many of the experiences that are widely considered to be traumatic, rape and sexual abuse being just two examples. The DSM III identified two characteristics distinguishing a traumatic event from other harmful experiences. The first is that trauma was seen to be an exceptional event "outside of the normal range of human experience." The second characteristic is the lingering presence of posttraumatic symptoms, which might range from nightmares and flashbacks to sleeplessness, distraction, and other symptoms of heightened physiological disorder. Typical traumatic reactions include the reliving of the event in dreams or in hallucinations, a preoccupation or obsession with retelling or reenacting the event, an inability to shake the feelings of vulnerability and shock that accompanied the initial injury, and a persistent sense of endangerment. Posttraumatic reactions can range from hypervigilance on one extreme to feelings of complete numbness on the other extreme.

The specification of traumatic experience as "outside human experience" has particular relevance for this discussion. As therapist Laura Brown points out, certain common types of human suffering, specifically those caused by incest or abuse, could not by this definition be considered traumatic (1995). Brown argues that what the courts and the diagnostic manuals took to be "human experience" was based on the normal life experiences of men of the dominant class. Consequently, such experiences as wartime injuries (both psychic and physical), sinking ships, and natural disasters were considered traumatic events, but daily, insidious, private experiences of oppression and abuse were not. Since 1994, with the publication of the DSM IV, the definition of trauma has been expanded so that traumatic events no longer need to be infrequent, unusual, or outside what Brown calls a "mythical human norm of experience" (1995, p. 111). Some writers on trauma have begun to speak of "insidious" and "daily" trauma to differentiate between different types of trauma (Root, quoted in Brown, 1995).

Kai Erikson claims that in order for the term trauma to be useful to us, we must resolve two terminological issues (1995). The first of these is a shift in emphasis from the actual trauma itself to the reaction to the trauma. It is, he says, "*how people react to them* rather than *what they are* that give events whatever traumatic quality they can be said to have" (1995, p. 185, original emphasis). The second is that trauma must be understood as resulting not only from a discrete happening, but "from a *constellation of life experience* . . . from a *persisting condition* as well as an acute event" (1995, p. 185, original emphasis). Erikson uses this definition of trauma to look at traumatized communities as different from assemblies of traumatized persons. While Erikson has worked with communities visited by natural disasters such as floods or earthquakes, his work has particular relevance for those who have endured slavery or the abuses of white supremacy. In the common vernacular, the term trauma is widely used to describe the effects of oppression. The words trauma and posttraumatic stress are used to designate a wide range of experience, even including the indirect experience of the children of Holocaust survivors and victims, for example.

Given the current interest in trauma studies within education, literary studies, and critical race theory, it is likely that official definitions of trauma will continue to broaden in response to this new political climate.[2] Consequently, it seems appropriate for this discussion to understand trauma in multiple ways: in the classic sense of an injury that continues to reinjure the wounded person; as the insidious and cumulative effects of oppression; as the aftermath of sexual or emotional abuse; and even as the collective memory of those who indirectly experience trauma, such as second-generation Holocaust survivors. Trauma has been passed on through generations of Native peoples torn from their homes, to Africans brought to the "new" world in slave ships and for the generations to follow, and trauma has been endured by people of all genders and races within the privacy of their homes.

Elliott's notions of racism and prejudice—and their antidotes—are grounded in the notion of insidious trauma. People of color in this culture experience daily indignities, abuse, and threats to their safety. If those who are oppressed in white supremacist culture must live with the pernicious and traumatic effects of prejudice day in and day out for all of their lives, Elliott's argument goes, then a small dose of such admittedly painful treatment administered to the privileged members of the culture is acceptable if it leads to the greater good of combating prejudice. Elliott's medical metaphors support this approach. Prejudice is the disease; her confrontational methods provide the inoculation that will bring about a "cure." Many who applaud Elliott's methods praise her on precisely these grounds:

> What Jane Elliott has done is to me no less significant than what Jonas Salk did with his polio vaccine in the 1950s. No longer need children's bodies be crippled by polio. Now we can prevent the crippling of their minds by racism. A teacher has shown us how. The only remaining question is whether we will *apply* the treatment—which consists, like the vaccine, of a tiny dose of the disease." (Peters, 1987, p. 172)

Elliott's Methods

Elliott promises her participants an experience that will be transformational. A one-time inoculation with the antiprejudice serum seems to hold out the promise of immunity for life. Numerous testimonials from previous participants dot Elliott's promotional materials. In *A Class Divided,* broadcast by PBS's Frontline in 1985, Elliott is reunited with her 1970 class as young adults, who describe the impact of their third-grade exercise on their lives. The video stands as a kind of testimony to Elliott's work, and is often cited as a longitudinal study of the impact of such teaching on student performance. While the inoculation metaphor implies the notion of a quick fix, the testimony of Elliott's students as depicted in *A Class*

Divided offers evidence that the effect of this exercise might in fact be quite long lasting. Elliott's students and their spouses talk candidly about the impact of the exercise on their lives, about their own commitment to not discriminating against others, and about how their participation as third graders in the Blue Eyes, Brown Eyes experience influenced them in raising their own children.

Confrontation takes the place of dialogue in Elliott's sessions. The single message Elliott means to deliver, in an unrelenting and sometimes brutal way, is this: As a white person, you have been privileged all of your life. To know what it feels like to be on the other side of the fence, you must be repeatedly humiliated, insulted, and silenced. There is no escape from this experience, just as there is no escape for people of color from the pernicious effects of racism.[3] Because there is no dialogue in Elliott's sessions, the possibility of moral agency on the part of her students is foreclosed. There is little space within Elliott's training sessions for white participants to replace their shame and guilt with moral commitments. When white participants attempt to claim some moral ground, or even to acknowledge their own privilege, Elliott clamps down on them or encourages other people in the audience to challenge them. Attempts at expressing moral agency are silenced in exactly the same way as defensive comments or challenges.

Elliott relies on a model of prejudice and oppression that implies a very simple notion of white privilege. Whites have power and privilege; people of color do not. While it is possible that it is precisely this clear and sustained focus on a single source of prejudice that has made Elliott effective in her work, as American culture becomes more and more diverse, and as the identities of American citizens blur in ever more complicated ways, it seems increasingly problematic not to explore multiple forms of oppression or make distinctions among forms of privilege. Elliott's tools are powerful, but they are also quite blunt. Her exclusive focus on racial prejudice overlooks the complex issues and ambiguous responses provoked by multiple forms of oppression and discrimination. Elliott does not admit, for instance, that skin color privilege may not protect a person from all forms of discrimination, nor allow for the possibility of conflict within communities of color or other marginalized communities.[4] Class and gender are only occasionally or indirectly invoked in Elliott's seminars, and indeed, Elliott has been criticized for her treatment of women.[5]

In her most recent video, *The College Eye*, Elliott introduces her session by talking about homophobia, sexism, ageism, and other sources of privilege and discrimination. However, having framed her talk in this broad way, Elliott then returns squarely to the issue of skin color privilege, outlining for her participants a hierarchy of suffering. Having badgered a young white woman for not bringing along a pencil and paper until the student begins crying, Elliott then challenges her. The exchange goes as follows:

ELLIOTT: "What are you crying about?" What are you crying about?
STUDENT: "My feelings were hurt."
ELLIOTT: "Why were your feelings hurt?"
STUDENT: "They just were."
ELLIOTT: "Should I feel sorry for her? Should I feel sorry for her? James Byrd, black man in Texas, dragged to death behind a pickup truck by three white males . . . I'm sorry, but those things happen because we live in a society in which people are allowed to treat those who are different badly simply because they are different. I cannot shed tears for a young, white female . . . I'm sorry, I have to save my sympathy and empathy for those who go through something much worse than this every day of their lives."

Later in *The College Eye*, Elliott repeats this strategy. When a second white female student begins crying, Elliott responds:

Martin Luther King, Jr. was shot. Are you in any physical danger here? Are you in any physical danger here? Is that girl in any physical danger? Emmett Till was hanged by his neck after he was beaten almost to death simply because he made a statement to a white woman.

We could debate whether it is politically productive to establish a hierarchy of suffering, and one could take issue with Elliott's treatment of her participants, who may themselves have suffered trauma in their lives, despite their skin color. But the broader question this raises for diversity work is how we might expand the discussion of diversity to address many different kinds of difference without diluting its impact and limiting its potential to bring about change.

Elliott seems to be working within an understanding of identity that is based on a simple binary logic of self and other. The self in her training sessions is constituted as a kind of surrogate victim, standing in for the other and briefly swapping identities: the oppressor becomes the oppressed. A more complex notion of identity would require an exploration of complexities and ambiguities, but there are no shades of gray in Elliott's classroom, no means to move beyond the simple binary of oppressor and victim other than this temporary, painful role reversal. It may well be this simple formula that makes Elliott so effective. Blue-eyed participants in her sessions cannot escape discrimination; once they are in the position of the victim, there is no opportunity for them to don the mantle of agency or power, even momentarily.

While Elliott's classroom space is created in service of liberatory goals, it is anything but a liberatory space itself. As bell hooks says, "education as the practice of freedom is not just about liberatory knowledge, it's about a liberatory practice in the classroom" (1994, p. 14). By contrast, much of Elliott's approach is deliberately and consciously oppressive. She engages in a bald exercise of power in the classroom, bullying her students, badgering them, humiliating them, and interrupting them as they speak. Surely this must bring discomfort to many participants of all races and ethnic backgrounds, if only by invoking their own prior experiences of abusive teachers, many of whom no doubt physically resemble Elliott.

Elliott's is a powerful message indeed, and while her approach is clearly effective in bringing home a lesson about discrimination, I believe we also need to continue to search for other ways to engage people in doing the difficult work of acknowledging and relinquishing privilege—ways that do not involve humiliation and pain for some, and rewards for others who publicly make a guilty admission of past blindness. Diversity trainers use many strategies to foster cultural awareness that are less traumatic than those Elliott employs. Writing strategies such as developing cultural autobiographies or defining terms such as culture, heritage, and ethnicity, viewing and discussing videos, reading and discussing works of fiction and nonfiction, and small group work involving role playing, scenarios, or discussions of first memories of difference, are just a few examples. Such experiences not only provide an opportunity for white participants to hear the experiences of people of color and begin identifying their own background and privileges, but they may also challenge people of color to listen more closely to those who are different from them. Many of these exercises are high risk, often provoking reflection and disclosure that may be quite traumatic for participants. While the terrible shock that comes with the recognition of privilege is an important first step in moving toward cultural competence, it is only the beginning of a lifelong process that must move beyond the initial painful realization of how one has been complicit in structures of oppression. Perhaps both time and trust are needed for this to occur. Some would argue that a liberatory classroom is one in which participants are treated with dignity and respect, and movement toward greater cultural awareness is fostered rather than inflicted. It is not a safe space that shies away from the expression of emotion, nor does it avoid confrontation. But perhaps it does not deliberately call forth feelings of humiliation, shame and fear on the part of some participants. Maybe it is a space in which trauma inevitably occurs, but is not deliberately inflicted by the instructor.

Elliott and Affirmative Action Pedagogy

The issues raised in this volume pose profound questions regarding who is being privileged and who is being protected by silencing, who benefits by incorporating cross-cultural dialogue into the classroom, and how power relations are revealed, masked or challenged by these practices.

In the essay introducing this collection, Megan Boler proposes affirmative action pedagogy as one response to racism in our culture. Boler suggests that it is an ethical imperative for instructors to silence voices in the classroom that express hostility toward traditionally marginalized groups:

> Until all voices are equal, we must operate within a context of historicized ethics which consciously privileges the insurrectionary and dissenting voices, sometimes at the minor cost of silencing those voices which have been permitted dominant status for the past centuries. (Boler, this volume, p. 13)

Boler describes a spectrum of affirmative action pedagogy based on how her colleagues in women's studies deal with expressions of "racist or homophobic ignorance." On one extreme is a faculty member who allows her students to express any views they wish. They are required to defend their opinions, which are then challenged by other participants in the class. On the other extreme is a professor who provides her students with a web site outlining what "areas of discussion, questions and remarks are not permissible" in her classroom. Both of these approaches fit within Boler's definition of affirmative action pedagogy, since ultimately they encourage previously marginalized voices to be heard.

Clearly, Elliott's motivation—to combat ignorance and battle prejudice—has much in common with affirmative action pedagogy. But because Elliott subjects her participants to a traumatic experience that is supposed to approximate the discrimination felt by people of color in American culture, her work provokes questions about the implications of silencing and controlling speech that are not easily answered within the affirmative action framework. It might even cause us to wonder under what circumstances abuse may be an inevitable outcome of silencing or controlling speech.

One important difference in Elliott's work is the deliberately intense emotional content of her training sessions. Elliott underscores the importance of this emotional pedagogy when talking of her experience with her Riceville third-graders:

> What I wanted to do was to make those sixteen third-graders aware of their effect on other people. I wanted them to live for one day as other people have to live for a lifetime. And if one day of pain helps them to refuse to inflict that kind of pain on even one other person during their lifetimes, then that one-day exercise was successful for that child. (Peters, 1987, p. 129)

And again:

> I think the reason it has lasted so long and has remained so strong is because it's something that they felt. . . . They internalized this experience. It's something that happened to their insides. It's not a lesson that was simply placed on them from the outside. It's something they experienced. (Peters, 1987, p. 130)

In her work with adults, it is not only the intense emotional content of Elliott's sessions that sets her apart, but also the parameters within which emotion is set up as raw experience inaccessible to rationality, reflection, or criticism.[6] As Boler points out, critical race theorists claim that rational dialogue will not change racist attitudes, because racism is irrational. Elliott's work as an antiracist educator seems to bear out this claim.

Elliott's pedagogical methods may separate her from Boler's affirmative action pedagogy even more strongly. Elliott's educational space is more theater than classroom, and it is anything but democratic. The only rules are those that she makes up, and they change as she goes along. Confrontation takes the place of discussion in her sessions. Only in the final segment of her workshops does Elliott engage in a kind of dialogue with her participants, which consists of Elliott posing questions to which her participants respond. Elliott maintains control of the discussion at all times, making this more of a question and answer session than a true dialogue. Only rarely does a member of the group challenge Elliott's statements.

Nonetheless, it is not easy to find alternatives to Elliott's work that have the power and impact of her sessions. It is clear that emotional pedagogy is an important component in diversity training, and it is also apparent that the expression of emotion in the university classroom is so strongly discouraged as to be nearly taboo. Students in most college classrooms seem emotionally deadened, and perhaps this is largely a result of prior traumatic educational experiences. In her essay in this collection, Ann Berlak describes a traumatic event that occurred in one of her classes, when an African American woman Berlak had invited to take over the class openly expressed her anger and rage. In a thoughtful and sensitive discussion of the events that transpired, Berlak shows us how both her students and she reached a higher level of awareness as a result of this incident. Berlak describes how the process of induction into the racial hierarchy leads to the severance of the connection between cognition and feeling, numbing the traumatized individual to injustice, and then goes on to demonstrate how her students were able to bridge this gap through their own expressions of anger and their thoughtful processing of the classroom event. And yet Berlak concludes her discussion by stating that such events cannot be the result of a strategy, but can only happen by accident.

Thus the paradox in Elliott's work remains unresolved: can we, like Elliott, ethically create traumatic episodes in order to provoke a deeper understanding? If not, what are the alternatives? Is it sufficient to be aware of the presence of trauma in the classroom, and to seek opportunities to foster—or simply not to stifle—traumatic experiences when we believe they will lead to deeper learning? Reflection on Elliott's work raises other important questions: How can we come to terms with the connection between pedagogy and pain? How are we to make sense of the relationship between emerging consciousness and psychic discomfort? Is it possible to find effective ways to teach about trauma without inflicting it—or without inflicting too much of it? Can we avoid repeating or perpetuating patterns of behavior that are part of the arsenal long used by those in positions of privilege? Having inflicted trauma on our students, how can we as instructors find or develop the skills we need to restore equilibrium or, to return to the question posed by Britzman, how can we "recognize and repair not just the harm done by others but the harm that occurs under the name of education?"

Notes

Thanks to Linda O'Neill for sharing many lively discussions with me about Elliott's work in preparation for our presentation at the Ohio Valley Philosophy of Education Society Conference, and to both Linda and Maureen McKnight for their thoughtful readings of this essay.

1. Elliott's videos are as follows: *The Eye of the Storm,* a 1970 ABC News documentary, depicts Elliott's experience with her third-grade class. *A Class Divided,* broadcast on the PBS Frontline series in 1985, dealt with the long-term impact of her 1970 exercise, reuniting her third-grade class. *Blue Eyed* was produced in 1996 by Denkmal Filmproductions; *Blue Eyed* shows a group of 40 Black, Hispanic and white teachers, police, school administrators and social workers in Kansas City. A California newsreel describes the video in this way: "The blue-eyed members are subjected to pseudo-scientific explanations of their inferiority, culturally biased IQ tests and blatant discrimination. In just a few hours under Elliott's withering regime, we watch grown professionals become despondent and distracted, stumbling over the simplest commands." *The Eye of the Beholder,* produced by Florida Public Television, dealt with adults and their reactions to discrimination. *The College Eye,* released in 2001 (originally with the title *The Angry Eye*) depicts Elliott conducting her "blue eyed" exercise with a group of college students. More recently, Elliott has released *The Stolen Eye,* which takes her "blue eyed" exercise to Australia, bringing Aborigines and white Australians together to talk about their country's history.

2. The publication of many recent works on trauma in various fields bears this out. In addition to those listed as references above are edited collections as follows: Belau & Ramadanovic's *Topologies of Trauma,* Miller & Tougaw's *Extremities: Trauma, Testimony and Community,* Simon, Rosenberg, & Eppert's *Between Hope and Despair: Pedagogy and the Remembrance of Historical Trauma,* as well as Farrell's *Posttraumatic Culture,* Silverman's *World Spectators,* and Cathy Caruth's *Unclaimed Experience: Trauma, Narrative, and History,* and *Trauma: Explorations in Memory,* to name only a few. Works on trauma are being published in many different fields, including psychology, history, sociology, philosophy, and literary studies.

3. There are participants who do choose to walk out of Elliott's training sessions, so perhaps this is not entirely true.

4. For instance, gay Asian American men often find themselves being "feminized" by other gay men of all races, thus suffering multiple forms of discrimination even within their own communities. Other examples are skin color discrimination within the black and Hispanic communities, and discrimination against those from other ethnic or racial backgrounds within communities of color.

5. Volk & Beeman (1998) did a gender-based analysis of *A Class Divided,* and they found that Elliott herself discriminated strongly in favor of the male students in her class, calling on them more often, responding more seriously to their comments, and so forth. They recommend using the video to teach about both race and gender.

6. My thanks to Linda O'Neill for this observation.

References

Belau, L., & Ramadanovic, P. (2002). *Topologies of trauma: Essays on the limit of knowledge and memory.* New York: Other Press.

Berlak, Ann. (This volume). Confrontation and pedagogy: Cultural secrets, trauma, and emotion in antioppressive pedagogies.

Boler, M. (This volume). All speech is not free: The ethics of "affirmative action pedagogy."

Britzman, D. (1998). *Lost subjects, contested objects.* Albany, NY: State University of New York Press.

Brown, L. (1995). Not outside the range: One feminist perspective on psychic trauma. In C. Caruth (Ed.), *Trauma: Explorations in memory* (pp. 100–112). Baltimore: Johns Hopkins University Press.

Caruth, C. (1995). *Trauma: Explorations in memory.* Baltimore: Johns Hopkins University Press.

Caruth, C. (1996). *Unclaimed experience: Trauma, narrative, and history.* Baltimore: Johns Hopkins University Press.

Cullen, P. (Director). (2002). *The stolen eye* [Motion picture]. San Francisco, CA: California Newsreel.

Erikson, K. (1995). Notes on trauma and community. In C. Caruth (Ed.), *Trauma: Explorations in memory* (pp. 183–199). Baltimore: Johns Hopkins University Press.

Farrell, K. (1998). *Post-traumatic culture: Injury and interpretation in the nineties.* Baltimore: Johns Hopkins University Press.

Golenbock, S., & Talmadge, W. (Producers). (2001). *The college eye* [originally entitled *The angry eye*] [Motion picture]. United States: Guidance Associates.

Herman, J. (1997). *Trauma and recovery.* New York: Basic Books.

hooks, b. (1994). *Teaching to transgress: Education as the practice of freedom.* New York/London: Routledge.

LaCapra, D. (2001). *Writing history, writing trauma.* Baltimore: Johns Hopkins University Press.

Leys, R. (2000). *Trauma: A geneology.* Chicago: The University of Chicago Press.

Miller, N., & Tougaw, J. (2002). *Extremities: Trauma, testimony and community.* Champaign, IL: University of Illinois Press.

O'Neill, L. All things with a reservation: The challenge of Alain Locke's critical relativism. Paper presented at 2002 OVPES conference, Dayton, OH.

Peters, W. (Director & Producer). (1970). *The eye of the storm* [Motion picture]. New York: ABC News.

Peters, W. (Director & Producer), & Cobb, C., & Peters, W. (Writers). (1986). *A class divided* [Motion picture]. Washington, DC: PBS Video.

Peters, W. (1987). *A class divided: Then and now.* New Haven, CT: Yale University Press.

Silverman, K. (2000). *World spectators.* Stanford, CA: Stanford University Press.

Simon, R., Rosenberg, S., & Eppert, C. *Between hope & despair: Pedagogy and the remembrance of historical trauma.* Lanham, MD: Rowman & Littlefield.

Strigel, C. & Verhaag, B. (Producers), & Verhaag, B. (Director). (1996). *Blue eyed* [Motion picture]. San Francisco, CA: Denkmal Filmproductions.

Volk, R.W., & Beeman, M. (1998, January). Revisiting *The eye of the storm:* The subtleties of gender bias. *Teaching Sociology,* 38–48.

Contributors

ANN C. BERLAK is an Adjunct Professor in the Department of Elementary Education at San Francisco State University. She is co-author with Sekani Moyenda of *Taking It Personally: Racism in Classrooms from Kindergarten to College* (Temple University Press, 2001). She has been teaching and reflecting on teaching for social justice for over thirty years.

MEGAN BOLER is an Associate Professor at Ontario Institute for Studies in Education at University of Toronto. She is the author of *Feeling Power: Emotions and Education* (Routledge, 1999) and her essays are published in a wide range of interdisciplinary journals, including *Cultural Studies, Women's Studies Quarterly,* and *Hypatia: Journal of Women and Philosophy.* Her research focuses on the media and communication studies, philosophy of technology, and social implications of cyberculture.

NICHOLAS C. BURBULES is Grayce Wicall Gauthier Professor in the Department of Educational Policy Studies at the University of Illinois, Urbana/Champaign. He has published widely in the areas of philosophy of education, technology and education, and critical social and political theory. He is also the current editor of *Educational Theory.* His forthcoming books include Gert Biesta and Nicholas C. Burbules, *Pragmatism and Educational Research,* and Michael Peters and Nicholas C. Burbules, *Poststructuralism and Educational Research,* both with Rowman and Littlefield Publishers, and due out in 2004.

SUZANNE DECASTELL is a Professor in Curriculum and Instruction at Simon Fraser University. Trained as a philosopher of education, she has devoted considerable effort to steering clear of its passenger section, instead stealing rides on its freight cars from the wrong side of the tracks. Her primary interest is in the epistemological impacts of traditional and new media, and she has tried hard to avoid ethics in its many insidiously moralistic forms. She has published widely and eclectically, and has edited three books.

INGRID M. ERICKSON is a multidisciplinary Ph.D. candidate at the University of Wisconsin—Milwaukee. Her research interests are in multicultural pedagogy, theories of emotion, and feminist, critical, and cultural theory. She is currently writing her dissertation on trauma and learning.

JIM GARRISON is a Professor of Philosophy of Education at Virginia Tech in Blacksburg, Virginia. His research interests center on pragmatism and education, especially the work of John Dewey. His work has been translated into many languages, including German, Italian, Russian, Portuguese, and Danish. His most recent book is *William James and Education* co-edited with Ronald L. Podeschi and Eric Bredo (Teachers College Press, 2002). Jim is a former president of the Philosophy of Education Society.

RONALD DAVID GLASS is a philosopher of education, currently an Associate Professor of Graduate Studies in the College of Education at Arizona State University West in Phoenix. He focuses on education as a practice of freedom, and on ideological formation and struggle in developing a just democracy. He has received numerous honors, including an Outstanding Teaching Award from the Stanford School of Education (1994), a Dondrell Swanson Advocate of Social Justice Award from Arizona State University (2000), and a Martin Luther King, Jr., Living the Dream Award from the City of Phoenix Human Relations Commission (2001). He has published in various journals, including *Educational Researcher, Studies in Philosophy and Education, Teacher Education Quarterly,* and *Reading Research Quarterly.*

BARBARA HOUSTON is a Professor of Philosophy of Education at the University of New Hampshire. She is a co-author of *The Gender Question in Education: Theory, Pedagogy & Politics* and has published articles on gender identity, feminist theory, ethics, and philosophy of education in such journals as *Hypatia: Journal of Women and Philosophy, Philosophy of Education,* and *Social Theory.*

ALISON JONES is an Associate Professor in the School of Education, University of Auckland, New Zealand. Her current research interests are varied, including cross-cultural pedagogy, Maori education in early New Zealand, and the effects on teachers of the social anxiety about touching children.

HUEY LI LI is an Associate Professor of educational philosophy at the University of Akron. Her areas of scholarship are ecofeminism, environmental ethics, and multiculturalism in the philosophy of education.

CRIS MAYO is an Assistant Professor in the Department of Educational Policy Studies and the Women's Studies Program at University of Illinois at Urbana-Champaign. Her research areas include sexuality studies, gender studies, and the philosophy of education.

Name Index

Subject Index